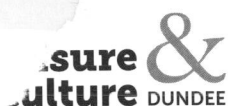
Laughing at Cancer

How to Heal with Love, Laughter and Mindfulness

Published by Brolga Publishing Pty Ltd
ABN 46 063 962 443
PO Box 12544
A'Beckett St
Melbourne, VIC, 8006
Australia

email: markzocchi@brolgapublishing.com.au

All rights reserved. No part of this publication may be reproduced, stored in a retrieval system or transmitted in any form or by any means electronic, mechanical, photocopying, recording or otherwise without prior permission from the publisher.

Copyright © 2017 Ros Ben-Moshe

National Library of Australia
Cataloguing-in-Publication data
    Ros Ben-Moshe, author.
    ISBN 9781925367843 (paperback)
    Subjects: Cancer--Patients--Australia--Biography.
              Cancer--Alternative treatment.
              Mental healing--Biography.
              Mind and body--Health aspects.
              Wit and humor in medicine.

Printed in Australia
Cover design by Alice Cannet
Typesetting by Elly Cridland
Photography by Daniel Letizi

BE PUBLISHED

Publish through a successful publisher. National Distribution, Dennis Jones & Associates
International Distribution to the United Kingdom, North America.
Sales Representation to South East Asia
Email: markzocchi@brolgapublishing.com.au

Laughing at Cancer

How to Heal with Love, Laughter and Mindfulness

Ros Ben-Moshe

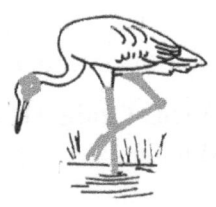

"Laugh at cancer... Really? Why would you do that? Simple really. When you laugh, there is no room for anything else. Laughter brings its own natural mindfulness that in turn brings our mind into connection with our body, and connects us joyfully with others. In doing so, laughter effortlessly transforms some of the darker emotions that can accompany cancer, enabling a deeper level of healing. So how do you laugh at cancer? Read *Laughing at cancer*! It's full of personal experience, useful facts and great tips. And the smile will come from deep within."

Ian Gawler OAM
Author of *Meditation - an In-depth Guide*
and *The Mind that Changes Everything*

"Being diagnosed with the big "C-word", CANCER, is discouraging. Still, the author of this book has found a couple other "C-words' to help her, and you, navigate that journey. Those words are "compassion" and "comedy." The former consisting of techniques in mindfulness and positive psychology and the latter which embraces life with laughter despite the disease. Filled with healing ideas, provocative questions, and lots of heart, this book is a must-read for anyone facing a life-challenging issue."

Allen Klein, MA, CSP
Author of *The Healing Power of Humor*
and *You Can't Ruin My Day*

"Standing back from and seeing the funny side of life, even cancer, can be profoundly therapeutic. It is for this reason that I suspect this book will be as healing for those who read it as it was for Ros Ben-Moshe who wrote it. Read it, cry and laugh, and, having read it, live every day with greater wisdom, passion and intention."

A/Prof. Craig Hassed MBBS, FRACGP
Mindfulness Coordinator, Monash University
Author *Mindfulness for Life*

"It is rare that a book has such a strong impact on my spirit. Ros describes her life-changing cancer journey so vividly, that I felt like I was right beside her every step of the way. Her journals transcend routine narratives and provide a powerful and poignant message of how one can find strength during the dreaded "C" diagnosis. Anyone living with chronic illness will benefit from the description of how a focus on positive energy can create healing techniques. Of special interest was how laughter became a form of mindful practice leading to her enhanced well-being. The creative questions at the end of each chapter stimulated additional personal insights. This book is a must read."

Mary Kay Morrison
Director Humor Quest. http://www.questforhumor.com/
Educator, Speaker, Author of *Using Humor to Maximize Living.*
President of AATH (Association for Applied
and Therapeutic Humor)

"This is a supremely captivating, inspiring, and penetrating book. Ros Ben Moshe explores the panoply of emotions that accompany a diagnosis of cancer, its treatment, and rehabilitation. She documents in engaging prose the process of coping with a universal vulnerability that affects millions of people around the world. The writing is exquisite, the story is powerful, and the message is compelling. This is more than a book about cancer. It is about how human beings can cope with frailties through laughter and love. The book will enrich your life and help you set priorities. Read it and recommend it to friends and loved ones. They will thank you."

Professor Isaac Prilleltensky
Author of *The Laughing Guide to Well-Being: Using Humor* and *Science to Become Happier and Healthier,* Dean School of Education and Human Development and Vice Provost for Institutional Culture, University of Miami.

"Ros Ben-Moshe has encapsulated the true meaning of 'laughter as medicine', demonstrating that even in your darkest moments you can choose to laugh and reap the health benefits of laughter. This book eloquently describes how when you laugh, you change and when you read this book your world will change as well."

Dr Madan Kataria
Founder Laughter Clubs Movement
Author of *Laugh for No Reason*

"An honest journal unfolds the daily truth of our lives with all its complexity--its interwoven strands making a whole. Sharing such truth is a generous gift. With her offering, Ros has revealed to us that laughter lightens the loads which we bear. She has reminded us of what we all once knew as children: laughter IS the very best medicine. Walking along Ros' way for a time may help each of us find our own."

Dr Rick Hayes
Former Head of the Department of Community Health,
La Trobe University, Melbourne, Australia.

"In time to come, the healing professions will conclude that belief, mind, attitude, and emotional mastery are the key ingredients for health and wellbeing. They will turn to this very approachable first-person read and point to Ros as being a prime example of how one person's determination to rise beyond victimhood of disease, contributed to recovery. If positivity is the doorway, and self-mastery the lock, then laughter is the key. If Ros does nothing else through this book than to inspire us to laugh at one's incipient and growing fear of the 'big C' then she will have contributed hugely to our wholeness and wellness."

Rabbi D. Laibl Wolf
Author of best-selling *Practical Kabbala* (Random House)
and Dean, Spiritgrow Wholistic Centre, Australia.

"Ros has bravely combined two human experiences that are usually on different ends of the spectrum we call life. And braver still, decided to share her very personal experiences so others can benefit from her insights. If you or your loved one is facing cancer, and you have an inkling that laughter, mindfulness, relaxation or even a smile could somehow help, this is the book for you. Certainly, laughing in such circumstances isn't easy, but not laughing doesn't make it any easier either. May you find some hope and inspiration through the words in this powerfully unique approach!"

Shamash Alidina
Author of *Mindfulness for Dummies*

Laughter is an untapped science. We didn't really know until now how to use it as a reliable therapeutic tool, but we do now and the results are amazing. In this book Ros Ben-Moshe takes you through her journey healing from cancer and the insights she gained along the way. Laughter is not the whole prescription, but she shows you how it made everything whole for her and how it can help you too. It's a message of hope and a valuable source of inspiration for people facing adversity."

Sebastien Gendry
Creator of the *Laughter Wellness* method

Acknowledgements

To my beautiful family: Danny, Josh and Zak. I penned this book fuelled by your love. You are my love, my light, my everything. I am so grateful that you are my family and from the bottom of my heart I thank you. To my extended family and friends — you complete my world. To the international laughter community, one word: Wow!

Special thanks to Josh for some wonderful creative writing input. To Heather Grant-Campbell, for critiquing my first draft — you are an absolute joy. To Bronwyn Roberts for the initial introduction to Brolga Publishing P/L. To the entire Brolga team: especially Mark Zocchi, Alice Cannet and Elly Cridland for the amazing editorial support and so much more.

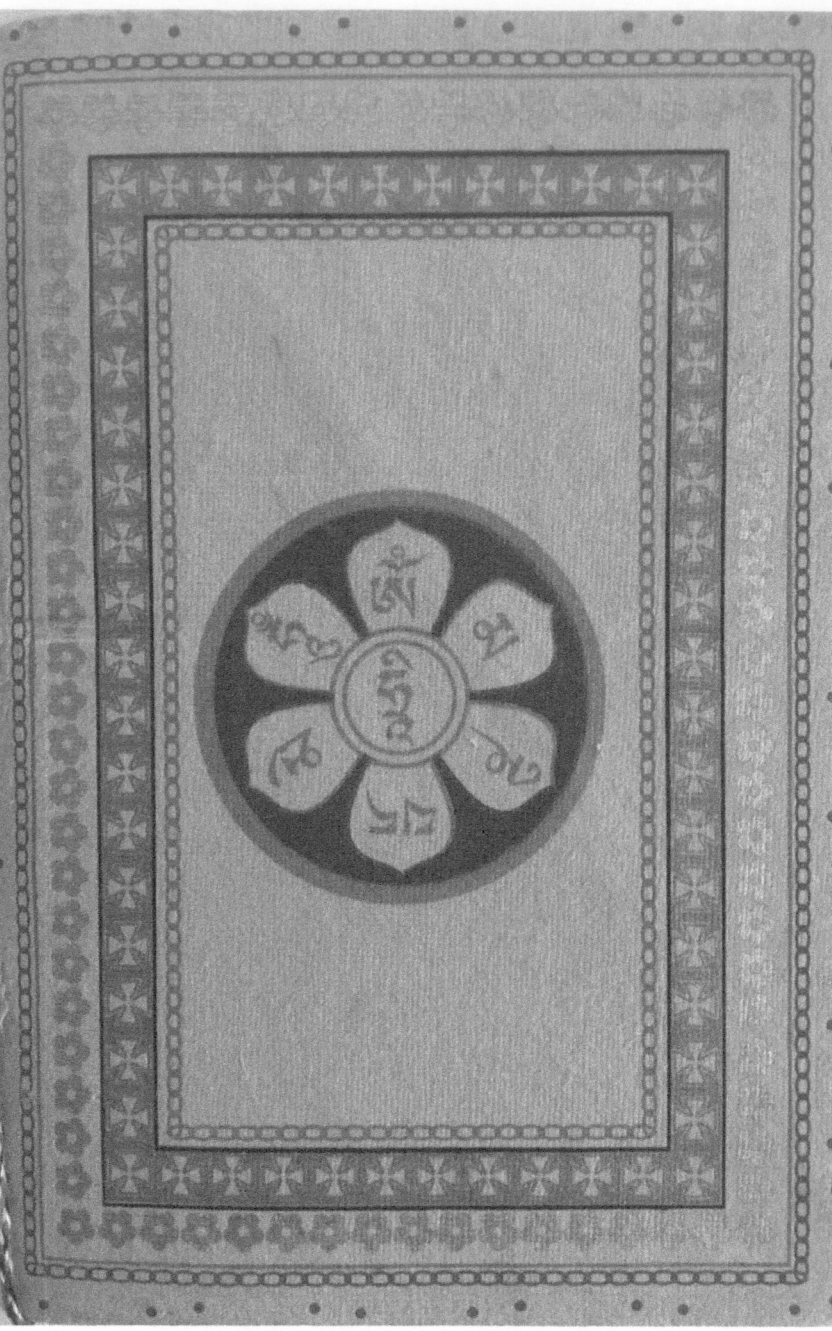

Introduction

Dear Readers,

Laughing at cancer, How to Heal with Love, Laughter and Mindfulness is is based on a series of journals I wrote following a shock diagnosis of bowel cancer days before my 43rd birthday.

Early into my writing I realised that as much as I was writing for myself I was also writing for other people who may be facing a significant health or life challenge. I aimed for my experiences and insights to assist and guide others on their own healing journey.

I share essential healing techniques, personal philosophies and professional insights as both a lecturer in health promotion and laughter wellness and mindfulness practitioner. Even though my experience was with bowel cancer, the healing strategies I employed in this book and much of what I went through are relevant to anyone living with a chronic illness or grappling with a significant life issue.

Laughter was integral to my journey to wellness. Not just laughter in the physical sense, but more broadly as a philosophy known as laughter wellness – a holistic practice positively orienting body and mind.

During this period of time my view of mindfulness expanded from that of a daily practice to a complete way of being. I derived so much benefit from daily mindfulness and experimented with different ways of sensing into and appreciating the present moment, far beyond any structured practice.

Increasingly I recognised laughter as a form of mindfulness: an anchor to the present moment. When you're laughing, you're laughing. It's very difficult to feel negative emotion. This is really important in terms of healing, as optimal healing occurs when less stress and tension resides in the body.

While surgeons and doctors attended to my physical condition, laughter, mindfulness and other positive psychology techniques enabled deeper healing. So even when circumstances may have appeared less than perfect, these helped align my mind and body to a state where optimal healing could occur.

I hope this book awakens your inner smile and leads you down a path of love, joy and life fulfilment. These philosophies profoundly transformed my life, and my wish is that they transform yours. I dedicate this book to your good health.

Wishing you much love, laughter and wellness,

♡ Ros Ben-Moshe

25 May 2011

This is where it all begins ... well it has to begin somewhere!

Now this isn't too hard, is it? I mean it's only taken ten thousand hints from the universe, a bowel cancer diagnosis and a lifetime of thoughts bursting the lining of my exploding head to finally begin to write, journal, download, do whatever it takes and in whatever manner it spills out.

The ink seals my words as testimony to a covenant I make with myself. From now on, all chatter cramming every nook and every cranny of my brain will have a place to go: my journal; a dedicated and devoted outlet where I can pour forth the depths of my unvocalised soul. It will soothe my mind and provide a resting place for my profound (and not so profound) thoughts, releasing any undesired and negative emotions that hibernate within. It will flow its own course. I am merely its conduit.

My life's journey has taken a new direction. A new current is pulling me, more forceful than ever before. There's no sitting back today and ignoring it. Tough decisions need to be made. Taking a deep breath in, I am considering what needs to be done. Countless people, too many, have been in similar situations before, far graver than mine. My brain is filled with opinions, facts and fear. I am unable to switch off. I am dreaming of the moment it heaves to a silent pause and rests.

I fear if it doesn't, my decision-making process will be encumbered, adding even more pressure to my pulsating head. I try tuning out the brain and tuning into my heart, gut and intuitive capacities, but they're just not communicating today. They are ensconced in their own battles. In this deafening noise

I can't find any inner silence or space to make sense of this.

Is this really happening to me? After all I am a health promotion consultant and laughter wellness facilitator. Surely that should somehow absolve me of poor health? I live and breathe wellness, don't I? I am considering the mind-body connection and wondering whether something, somewhere along the way has caused a conjunction between seamed parts. I have tried to think positively. I really have done my best. So why then have I had so much sickness? Chronic fatigue syndrome (CFS), parasites, shingles, a Deep Vein Thrombosis (DVT) and now this malignant polyp: a mere 21mm in diameter, with a few pesky cancerous cells outside of its margin. It's hard to believe something so small can amount to something as life-changing as this. 'This can't be happening to me,' screams over and over in my head making me woozy. I will an out-of-body experience to free me from my own—not that I've ever had one!

Another solitary breath in and out, slow and deep. Time to close my eyes and contemplate my next step both in the written and physical worlds. Nothing makes sense. I wish I could stop thinking so much. The more I write, the more real it feels, and that is the last thing I want. I am too distraught to contemplate sleep. I pray that after I give in to sleep, I'll wake up and today's nightmare will have been just that.

30 May 2011
What do you want from me?

Sometimes the burdens of life mount like a pressure cooker, exploding its lid and bursting with contents. Have I not had enough life lessons? Do I really need more? Apparently yes, and with a little added resistance. It just goes to show that when you think you know it all—or at least appear to be heading in the right direction—there's still a blind spot. You can never know what's in store for you. We're just pawns in a metaphysical chess game where those in the heavens above already know the outcome; yet we remain blissfully ignorant.

Yesterday I experienced one of the greatest ironies in my life. As I stirred from slumber to woken consciousness, a tear cascaded slowly down my cheek, shed in the realisation I was no longer sleeping. This was not a bad dream but my new reality. Oh the irony: I had finally landed a dream job, an amazing opportunity, a small amount of financial security, and a bit of prestige. There might even be champagne. In fact, there would definitely be champagne upon signing the contract for my new job; or at least this was how it had played out in my mind after receiving the job offer two weeks ago. Well, that champagne ending morphed into a particularly sombre birthday in the relatively short history of Rosalind Jennifer Holsman.

Today is the deadline to sign and return my declaration for the permanent position of part-time lecturer at La Trobe University in yet another irony: Public Health and Health Promotion. Instead of the anticipated birthday lunch with friends, I had a midday appointment with a surgeon. This was no run-of-the-mill consultation, it was life-changing and I was considerably under-prepared.

How can it be that in less than two weeks, I've gone from a routine appointment with my GP where I once again aired my frustrations about my irritable bowel, to a colonoscopy and gastroscopy, and finally to this? Sitting opposite the surgeon with my soulmate and life partner of 25 years, Danny, numb and too terrified to speak or move.

Ever since a parting gift of a Giardia parasite from a family holiday in Thailand, I've grown used to the occasional sight of blood and mucous in my stools, finding it more annoying than alarming. My naturopath thought I'd probably picked up another parasite, which made sense as a stool test around 12 months ago had returned normal. What else could it be?

Following my colonoscopy less than a week ago, I left the recovery room, the gastroenterologist's words still fresh in my ears, 'You're one lucky woman. I removed a polyp from your bowel but it all looks fine.'

Five days later, an unexpected phone call summoned me back to his consultation suite. As soon as I arrived, I exclaimed, 'You said it looked fine. Are you sure?' Our eyes met but I lost focus. Then the barrage of thoughts and questions jumbled amidst the many hushed expletives. What am I going to tell my parents? This is the last thing they need. What about our two beautiful boys aged 12 and 15? I pushed away that thought as far as my conscious mind would allow. It was too painful.

I'm sure the poor gastroenterologist wished his next patient would pound on the door demanding his immediate attention. 'So does this mean you remove a little bit more of the area around the polyp?' I asked. Wary of sending my doting husband and myself into even deeper shock, he kindly suggested we discuss surgical options another time. OK, maybe it wasn't as bad as I feared, but then why the grave look? Curiosity got the better of me, and as we were both glued to our seats I asked what the next steps were. I sank deeper and deeper into the seat feeling smaller and more insignificant than ever before.

I didn't have to undergo a full bowel resection, he explained. I could instead opt for a partial resection but there would be no way of knowing for certain whether the cancer had spread. cancer? What? This was just a tiny polyp! I didn't have cancer. This was a malignant polyp. Full stop.

Any trace of blood in my face now drained away as my heart pumped harder and harder trying to escape the sinister truth. The next piece of news, the piece de resistance, came fast: the only way to test if the cancer had spread to the lymph was to do a full bowel resection. Danny and I had clearly both misunderstood. How could it be that, with all the advances of modern medicine, navigating around the bowel to the lymph wasn't an option? Surely a high or even low-tech medical apparatus had been developed for just this reason? How seemingly 'third-world' to have to cut through the bowel! I had heard about friends who'd had breast cancer and even though testing the lymph nodes was traumatic, it was a relatively straightforward procedure.

I cautiously asked if he thought the cancer might have spread; yet as soon as these words left my mouth, my inner voice piped up, 'Don't ask a question you really don't want to know the answer to.' But it was too late. They had escaped along with more expletives. He said he really didn't know and would refer me to a highly regarded colorectal surgeon who would be able to answer my questions and perform any subsequent surgery.

This was much bigger than I feared.

His words spun out of control in my head and kept spinning for two days until we landed in the here and now, long-faced in the said surgeon's office on my 43rd birthday.

After the formal introductions a diagram was placed in front of us with a small circle highlighting the polyp in my rectum. Given its size the surgeon estimated there was a 3–5% chance that the cancer had spread but he wouldn't know until further investigation. I felt marginally comforted. That didn't seem too high. I mean, what's 3%?

He continued talking while Danny and I sat in a state of paralysis incapable of uttering a single syllable, let alone a full sentence. Because the surgical site was so low in the bowel, the surgeon matter-of-factly informed us I would need a new rectum, which he would construct. Moreover due to poor circulation in the region I would be fitted with a temporary ileostomy. An ileostomy? What the hell was that? I had heard of a colostomy but that was for really old people.

I recapped the main points in my head: a new rectum, an ileostomy, and the removal of a ruler's length of bowel. A five-hour procedure for the bowel resection and a two-hour operation to reverse the ileostomy three months down the track—if all went well and I was not left with a permanent bag. The recovery from the first operation would take around eight weeks and the side effects included the alteration or potential loss of sexual function as well as forever altered bowel function.

Feeling utterly demoralised, I stormed out of the surgeon's office (as politely as I could). I was brimming with resolute defiance mixed with fury, rage and a strong shot of denial; but I knew one thing for certain: there was absolutely no way I would ever have a full bowel resection.

First stop thereafter was the local bottle shop where we hastily purchased two bottles of hard liquor: the first, vodka with acai berries and pomegranate (how exotic and with a wellness twist), the other, a Black Label whisky. I wasn't going to scrimp on price or quality today of all days. Both these beverages hold spiritual and religious attributes for a l'chaim (to life) and I was not sure whether to go Hasidic or Polish for extra l'chaim potency. Safe to say I sealed the day's fate with vodka for added nominal health attributes. As for the contractual champagne, it was left corked.

The lingering on the 'Declaration of injury/illness' contractual page soured what two weeks ago had been elation, at a time when little attention had been paid to the small print. Surely it is a good sign though to complete and return this permanent work contract by close of business on such a sombre and surreal birthday?

What was the best birthday you ever celebrated and what made it so special?

....

....

....

In general do you make a point of celebrating good life events? What was the last thing you celebrated and in what way?

....

....

....

Make yourself a promise right now to always celebrate life's special events.

3 June 2011

When you know what to do

On occasions through life's passage, one is confronted with seemingly unsolvable challenges, dilemmas and angst.

Journeying into the foray of the C-word—I just can't bring myself to write this word in full—is one of those occasions. You don't always have enough time on your side to fully flesh out, research and come to a decision, free from wrangling internal and external voices.

Just three days ago, my head imploded as the left and right hemispheres of my brain argued and competed with each other to reach a consensus. How could I ever make such a tough decision? Why did I have to make it in the first place? How would I know if I made the right choice?

As luck would have it I was alerted to a timely two-day workshop, Health, Healing and Wellbeing, run by Dr Ian Gawler AM, founder of the Gawler Foundation Cancer Institute and author of *The Mind that Changes Everything*.[1] Steeped in sorrow I drove to the 'cancer domain'. I was clearly seated in the 'bowels side' of the hall. On my left sat a middle-aged man who'd had full-on bowel cancer resulting in chemo and the works, and on my right was a youthful-looking woman who'd had a bowel resection following the mysterious dying of part of her colon. Hearing other people's stories made me swiftly realise I had much to be grateful for.

There was a lot to take in, but what flagged my attention was how to make a decision that would avoid or reduce any potential regret. For this, I needed to be in a clear state of mind, full of

---

1   Gawler, I., The Mind that Changes Everything, Brolga Publishing,

commitment and enjoyment, and absolve the need to question, perhaps six months down the track, if the right decision was made. In other words, I should avert the 'what ifs' slippery slope. In my current state, the enjoyment aspect seemed rather impossible. I mean, how can you enjoy something so difficult? But I promised to give it a go.

Several other points screamed at me, but one in particular made its way to the forefront of my mind now dulled by information overload. Who would be on my internal decision-making committee? How could I broaden my support network, not just on a physical level, but also spiritually? Who could invoke a higher power, not necessarily God, but something or someone who inspires me or gives me strength? Immediately my Rabbi's kind face, framed by a cotton wool beard and wise eyes deep as wells, came to mind. A world-renowned leader of Jewish spirituality and mysticism, he had always been a source of comfort and inspiration whose aura somehow emanated a closer connection to God. I would contact him.

Feeling considerably more empowered I returned home to face one of the bloodiest battles my mind had ever waged. I considered the casualties and fallout. In most battles, there are no true winners but there are always losses. Stakes can be high and strategies complex and risky, but at the end of the day, one strategy triumphs over another. Not all casualties are bad. Calculatedly I weighed up the pros and cons. I sat with them, cogitated, debated and wrestled with them. I wanted to escape my body and absolve personal responsibility by letting someone else make this decision. I wanted to run and keep running. After some time, I realised I was in a position of strength, able to choose the path I would follow. This was something to be grateful for. I decided to farewell negativity, toxicity and stale energy and chose the option I had initially and emphatically rejected: to have a full bowel resection.

As I write this, the consensus I've reached leaves me feeling an all-pervasive, almost disquieting sense of peace. I can't quite believe how sweet this victory feels; lightness consumes me as the lead weights and seismic forces are dismantled. This is the 'ah' moment: realising what I need to do to ensure the best possible outcome, not only for my physical health, but also for my spiritual and emotional wellbeing. The deafening inner chatter has been silenced. Like the calm after a tidal wave, or a blue sky reclaiming its place after a torrid, cloudy storm, I am at peace. Whatever is in store for me, I know I will not regret my decision. At the end of the day it is my decision, not the surgeon's, not Danny's, but mine alone.

Conscientiously I am going to refer to my current situation as 'challenging' rather than 'bad'. It's just not a matter of bad or good. It is what it is, and even though I have not consciously chosen it nor would I ever want to, inspiration, growth and positivity will germinate. I will triumph over this challenge and take heed of the fundamental lessons inextricably bound within it. I will rid myself of the old, choosing surgery as the best means to attain optimal health potential.

In order to be free, a full bowel resection is my only real choice. I know how uncertainty would play out in my body; the fear of something lurking in some form or other would indubitably wreak emotional and physical havoc. It would destroy me. I would live in a state of constant fear, listening out for a bomb ticking away, unconsciously awaiting detonation. I am taking no chances. I need to know with 100% certainty that no cancerous cells linger beyond my bowel's lining.

I am guided by Ian Gawler's wise words, 'Make a decision for the right reason, stick with it, enjoy it, and don't look back.' Now there is no room for looking back. I am free of the shackles of indecision. This is true individual empowerment. These are the real freedoms we are blessed with: the freedom not only to choose, but to respond. Do we accept it wholeheartedly, without regret, NO exception? Or do we partially relent from a perspective of desperation, futility or limited hope?

In addition to the full bowel resection I will also investigate the best possible means of achieving full healing. From my current vantage point, this seems to be meditation. If only I had reached out to it in a more meaningful sense before. Sure I've dabbled with it, but I now understand that's not enough. It has to be a scheduled ongoing event used as a tool to restore my health, my life and my wellbeing. I need to tether myself to it: to breathe, imbibe and co-habit with it. I need to shape my days around it, rather than haphazardly squeeze it between other stuff, of which there is always guaranteed to be plenty.

I will begin today. I will continue tomorrow and the days thereafter. I will use meditation as a form of catharsis to support me through any anxiety prior to my surgery and assist subsequent healing and recovery. I will meditate to restore wavering vitality levels, so swamped by lethargy, and so deep that my body assumes them as its normal set point.

I am feeling the potential to be reborn; optimism is well within reach. I am opening my heart to spirit and warmly inviting it into my entire being. I must not be scared or weighed down by burdensome fears. I must open the door to my potential, to my power, to the inner force whose pulse I am beginning to feel reawaken within me. I must not be afraid as I have felt the love and support of the universe.

I will be nurtured and guided back to the path of wellness. I don't need to rush. The first step has already been taken; this is always the most difficult one. I am contemplating a baby's first tentative steps: a huge milestone that in no time is taken for granted and forgotten as we journey onto a life filled with millions of taken-for-granted steps.

Let's pause for a moment to relive the wondrous excitement and participation of our very first physical step. Then take some time to celebrate each and every first step (beyond the physical) that we have taken, to get us to where we are now.

Have you ever received life-changing information and made a promise to yourself to do something to improve your wellbeing?

....
....
....

Did you adopt a new wellbeing practice?

....
....
....

If not, can you think of something you can do right now that would benefit your wellbeing? Ask yourself why you haven't already been doing it.

....
....
....

Don't put it off any longer.

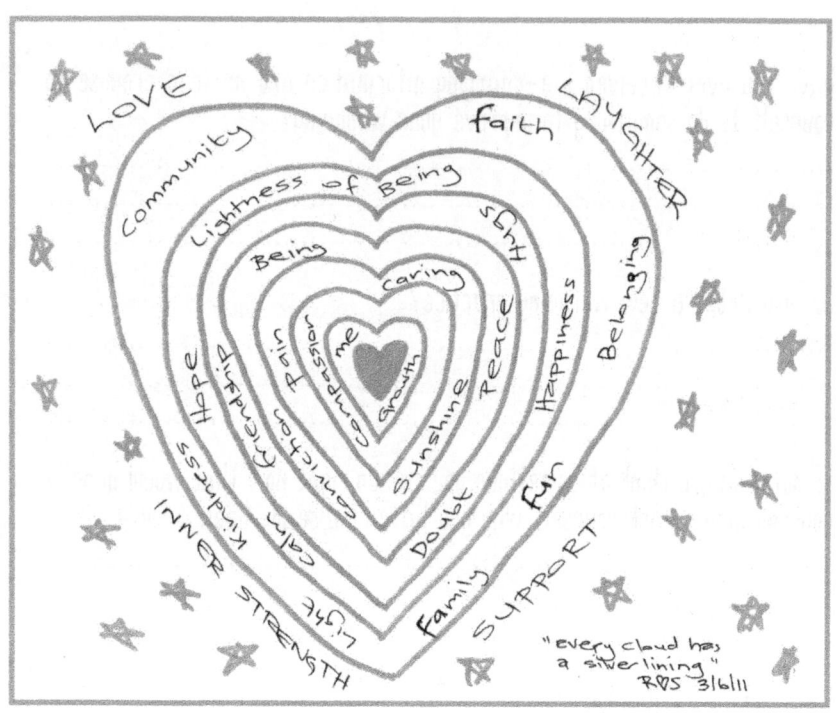

4 June 2011

My Dream

The night after making this mammoth decision I had the most vivid dream, an exquisite guide preparing me for what lay ahead. As remarkable as the dream was, its clarity struck me even more. I don't usually recall my dreams, and if I do, it's only vaguely and momentarily.

I am standing at the top of a mountain in the beautiful Red Hill region in the hinterland of the Mornington Peninsula, Victoria. Ahead of me is a sign to Amanda's Art Gallery—Amanda is a dear friend and transformational healer who lives in Israel. We lost contact and have not seen one another in more than a decade. I don't want to get distracted as I know I have to get to my beautiful boys, Josh and Zak, who are all alone on a nearby mountain.

Ahead I see a firebreak down the mountain. The pine stumps are about a foot high and painted white. It is a very steep path and looks quite daunting, but instinctively I know this is the quickest and best way forward.

Lying flat on my back I begin gliding my way down, comfortably skimming the stumps yet not really feeling any discomfort. About two thirds of the way down I pass through a thick cloud of swarming insects. They bite me, making me itchy and irritated. Their grouping is so dense I think I will never pass through them; darkness is all around. But just as it had appeared out of nowhere the swarm soon begins dissipating, and finally disappears save for one or two odd insects.

The path ahead is clear and I continue gliding down the firebreak relatively unencumbered until I am reunited with Josh and Zak. All is well! Our relief in seeing one another is palpable. Emotions run high as we embrace and share multiple hugs.

I have never felt so scared, but I am out of the woods!

Can you recall a dream you had relating to a significant moment or event that was prophetic in some way?

....

....

....

During times of angst have you ever made a conscious wish before you sleep for a dream to help guide you? If not, why not experiment? As our analytical minds are put to sleep, dreams open the door to one's unconscious mind and perhaps even to a spiritual realm.

6 June 2011

Forced Laughter

Today I held a laughter session for the annual party of a lingerie company, of all places. At the time of booking I was thrilled to receive an invitation to present to a new client, certain it would be a fun crowd. For the past few days all I have wanted to do was cancel. How could I muster the strength and state of mind to run a laughter session when all I wanted was to hide from the public and cry? This was undoubtedly the LAST place I felt I could be.

My mind casts back to the first time I was introduced to Laughter Yoga at a World Health Promotion conference some five years ago. So entranced by this delightfully wacky practice, not long thereafter I trained as a laughter yoga leader. Still fresh in my mind was my first official laughter gig for local residents at a community health centre. I had been told to expect a crowd of around ten. Grey hair and wrinkles was all I saw as six septuagenarians trickled through the door. Burying my disappointment I began the session. Barely moments passed before bright eyes, youthfulness and a spark for life reclaimed the room. Boy had I underestimated this crowd and the power of laughter. As they say the rest is history. Until this moment in time I have delighted in facilitating laughter yoga sessions on the side of my academic life. Yet come this morning, I am feeling distinctly less than delighted. Too late to cancel, I made myself presentable, psyched myself up and garnered as much energy as my night of sleep deprivation allowed. I put on a face and not just the makeup kind! If there was a measure for stress, mine was stratospheric.

Thirty or so chatty and excitable ladies filled the room. Their energy was palpable whilst mine still had not entered the room. The hostess introduced me, saying, 'We're so happy to have Ros here today, especially as she is going through a bit of a tough time at the moment.' I had previously forewarned the hostess I was in the midst of a mini health crisis, but had not imagined she would divulge this to the audience. Her words were the last thing I wanted to hear. Please tears stop welling up!

I took a deep breath in and focused on the task ahead. I explained how laughter yoga evolved decades ago in India, and more recently had taken the world by storm through laughter clubs, with Indian Doctor Madan Kataria[2] and his wife Madhuri at the helm. As it doesn't rely on humour to be effective it is a winning formula that can be used for people, such as yours truly, who really are not in the mood to laugh. Combining laughter exercises, deep breathing and clapping whilst chanting 'ho, ho, ha ha ha,' I went on to explain that laughter being used as medicine or therapy was not new – far from it. As far as back the 1500s one particular Court jester is believed to have kept Queen Elizabeth 1 in better health than her physicians. In more modern times clown doctors in over-sized shoes and bulbous red noses traipse down hospital corridors around the world bringing play, humour and laughter to patients, family and staff. There's an array of humour based laughter therapy and non-humour based laughter therapy: the common denominator being laughter for health's sake.

It's not just the feel good nature of laughter; there is the hard-core science behind it. I then recounted some of the many health benefits including its ability to trigger endorphins (those happy hormones), to stimulating the immune and lymphatic systems, improving circulation, reducing pain and muscle tension and even lowering blood pressure.

I asked the group how many times a day on average they laughed; a question I'm sure they would never have thought about before, let alone been asked. I then had them guess how many times a day children laugh on average. Everyone was amazed to

2   Kataria, M. Laughter Yoga International http://laughteryoga.org, 1999

hear how often that was in comparison to adults. I invited their contributions and a lively discussion ensued. Unsurprisingly stress topped the list, with one lady bellowing, 'children don't have mortgages!' I relayed my own theory: children laugh from the heart; they don't think about it, they just do it.

I was saved from having to draw on precious grey matter having given this spiel countless times before and reverted to autopilot. I relayed how, in most societies, as we grow older, our laughter-self becomes conditioned, beginning as early as our junior school years when teachers scald us for laughing out of turn. No one likes to be told off. Just as no one likes to be laughed at. All too soon we learn the harsh distinction between laughing with someone and laughing at someone. Over time this intensifies, as we become increasingly conscious of how others perceive us when we laugh. How will we be viewed if we laugh seemingly inappropriately or excessively? The professional workplace is the biggest culprit. Our inner voice decrees, 'I'm in a serious job now it can't look like I'm having too much fun or people will assume I'm not doing my job well.' Rather than just laughing for laughter's sake as we did as children, we bring an intellectual or critical quality to our laughter, so for many, over time, the laughter-fountain dries up. We laugh on the inside, saying things like 'that's really funny', and far too often abstain from laughing out loud.

I refrained from getting too bogged down in technicalities, battling far worse than brain-fog, but as a pedlar of hope, I wanted to recount some basics of neuroplasticity: the brain's amazing ability to change and heal itself in response to mental experience.

Captive audience in hand, I delivered the exciting news that the brain is not as fixed and unchangeable as was once thought. As I write, I clearly recall the relief I first felt when exposed to these notions in Dr Norman Doidge's book, *The Brain That Changes Itself* [3]. His research discounted the misconception I had lived with my whole life: that all those collective bumps and knocks to my head had NOT resulted in permanent brain cell loss. We

---

3   Doidge, N., The Brain That Changes Itself, James H. Silberman Books, 2007
(Scribe Australia 2008)

can grow new ones. We can rewire our brain to open new neural pathways with infinite potential. The more we do something in a particular way the more it becomes automatic, creating a new neural pathway or strengthening an already existing one.

Relaying this critical point, a few blank looks prompted me to illustrate by way of example. Given the crowd, what first came to mind was something to do with a bra, but as I couldn't conceive of a different way of fastening the strap's hooks, that example fumbled before it even began. Mindful of time marching, my next thought was to someone who always wore their watch on their left arm, but for whatever reason decides to start wearing it on their other arm. Then over a period of weeks the placement of their watch on their right arm becomes automatic. Far more exciting than a reorientation of a watch is our ability to rewire our brain to positive thinking.

I chimed it's about being mindful and bringing a conscious level of awareness to smiling and laughter. The more we choose to smile and laugh, the better worn those neural pathways become, so the default response from perhaps a grimace or even the absence of response becomes laughter or a smile. Then I grinned out my elevator pitch as my face, like porcelain, felt like it would crack: smiling and laughing more often rewire the brain to a complete and constant state of calm, joy and awareness.

I posed one final question hoping to mop up any remnants of inner or outer critique. 'Is a jog on a treadmill any different from a jog around the park, aside from the physical environment?' If you laugh with the right intention—choosing to laugh—then there really is not much difference. When you laugh, you receive all the wonderful health benefits even if the initial stimulus is simulated. Moreover, the contagious nature of laughter is, on our side, manufacturing real or involuntary laughter—the type that leaves you gasping for air. The non-verbal track in my mind was, 'If I can fake it 'til I make it the way I feel today, then you most definitely can!'

They were rearing to go and for comfort's sake I suggested we move into the garden. I was hoping the neighbours wouldn't mind peals of laughter permeating the glorious mid-afternoon sunshine.

As we proceeded outdoors I was still carrying some resistance for the actual laughter part of the session, with a hidden urge to run and hide, but the front door was in the opposite direction.

Thankfully, this group was no different to any other I had led, and in no time at all, splutters and guffaws of laughter could not be restrained. They were lapping it up, as was I. My 'stressometer' went right down. I couldn't feel any stress at all. I was lost in laughter.

After the session I asked people to share how they felt: happier, lighter, brighter, less anxious or stressed, more or less tired, warmer or cooler. I was delighted to hear that they too felt happier lighter, brighter and less anxious and stressed. I was decidedly more enlivened. My circulation had rebooted as warm blood effortlessly flowed to my extremities. For the first time in weeks I felt an excitement for life, for really living.

I am so grateful to have been forced to laugh. I certainly wouldn't have otherwise, well at least not in such an intense and concentrated fashion. Even now, several hours later, I'm weightless, freed of the lead weights that had ascended after my diagnosis. Powerful stuff!

I am wondering when I will lead my next laughter session and in what state I will be. My gut tells me it won't be for a while; so long may today's laughter-effect endure.

XXXX

During stressful times have you tried something to shift from your darkened mood? If so, what have you done?

....

....

....

One of the quickest and most effective ways to achieve this is through laughter or with a smile. If this does not happen naturally, try thinking about something funny or someone who makes you feel good about yourself. A genuine heartfelt smile can change your whole physiology as endorphins (happy hormones) are released. Why not try one now?

8 June 2011

Shhhh...hush...

It just dawned on me I am the source of awkward silence. The hushed conversations and disquiet in the air.

How can it be that in the course of two weeks, things that were always talked about are now not? Conversations feel fraudulent; there's no hint of normalcy. How can there be any when chats begin in such forced fashion? No one dares air their own troubles or concerns. General chitchat and everyday complaints are absent. In this moment, everyone else's lives seem a picture of perfection. I am now living in what feels like a surreal experiment.

Never one for small talk, my inner resistance is growing; that, and the tears quickening their pace, edging me dangerously close to flooding point.

I think of the times I've been privy to these types of conversations and imagine the non-verbalised track in people's shocked minds: 'I can't believe it.' 'Have you heard?' 'So young.' 'cancer? Really?' 'She seemed so healthy.' 'Oh no...how terrible.'

Yet there have also been times since I was co-opted on this roller-coaster ride, I have almost felt psyched, as if higher forces had chosen me to serve the 'Greater Good'. I am aware this may sound deluded—or taking positive thinking to an extreme—but in the end I know I will be a stronger person for this. I will triumph. I will learn. I will grow. I will rise to the occasion, give back, nurture, and I will heal. My body will be rid of any lingering toxins and replenished by Vitality and Spirit: the true essence of life.

Will it be easy? Probably not. Will it be achievable? Yes, because I've made a commitment to myself to live, really live. Not half-heartedly, or casually, but with a bolstered level of commitment that often comes when faced by life's ephemeral nature. I'm certain that if I searched Google for 'let's really live' support groups, activities such as jumping out of airplanes would come up; not the answers I am looking for. Yet it does get me thinking, what does living really entail? My hunch is it's about all the minutiae things that compose your day. Not the big life events you have to wait for half a lifetime in the hope you will then reap the rewards.

So in the days ahead I'm going to embrace the recommendations by Positive Psychologist Dr Barbara Fredrickson, to create micro moments of joy that lift my spirit, boost and enlighten my happiness and enrich my soul. I need to identify things that make my heart sing. These need to be ritualised. Whilst some activities such as grocery shopping, washing clothes and keeping the house in a semblance of order may need to be done, they should be recognised for what they really are: chores that are rarely filled with joy or purpose. At this time especially I need to enhance my joy and actualise a greater sense of meaning and purpose.

And with that I'm signing off, resting my weary eyes and body to rejuvenate with a nice, transformational, deep slumber.

X

List 5 things that make your heart sing.

....
....
....

List 5 things that often get in the way.

....
....
....

10 June 2011

Why can't it be the 'little c' instead?

The language around cancer really riles me. It's all-pervasive: 'she had cancer', 'he had cancer', as opposed to being contained and specific, for example, she had a cancer, he had a cancer. Saying a person has cancer creates a misperception that a person's whole body, as opposed to a contained, specific area, is cancerous. Whilst in a minority of cases, if someone has terminal cancer (i.e. it has spread to the point of no containment) this may be true, in the majority of cases, it isn't.

It's time to change the default language around cancer. Acknowledging someone has a cancer is far more empowering than saying she or he has all-consuming cancer. The same can be said about other conditions. Referring to a person 'with a disability' as opposed to 'disabled', or who 'has diabetes' instead of 'diabetic', emphasises and empowers the healthy part of that person. It focuses on the areas that are functioning well rather than the sickness. In my case, and all being well, this will be just a small malignant pocket within the bowel.

It's an important clarification and one I wanted to impart to the boys. So this afternoon, having decided on my course of action, we held a family meeting. Seated around our dining table, I downplayed the potential seriousness of my situation, explaining, 'I have a small polyp in my bowel and a few of the cells in and around it have some cancerous cells. It should be fine, but just to be on the safe side, I am having a larger operation. It's a very big operation, and for a while it will appear like I'm sicker than I really am.'

We steer clear of statistics, allaying chaos and fear, navigating instead towards hope and stability. We sidestep the 'what ifs', deciding that if they ask, we will then respond. The subtext is very clear: 'Mum does not have the Big C, a small part of her bowel does!'

The last thing I want and fear they will hear is, 'Your mum's got cancer.' With the menacing grapevine dangerously encroaching we tell them people may jump to conclusions, not fully understanding my situation. One of my friends has already enthusiastically offered to go wig shopping with me, making my natural hair well and truly stand on end.

Containing the cancer to a specific body part enables the rest of my body to be in a state of well-being, optimising healing. Succumbing to an overall diagnosis of cancer dilutes the healing effect, weakening my whole self. The more harmonious and positive my state of mind, the better.

We will deal with the mountain if it presents itself; at the moment it's a rather large and inconvenient molehill—to put it mildly. It's breaking down the 'too hard basket' into wicker strands. It doesn't diminish the huge ramification of a cancer diagnosis, which no semantics of language can change, but it does relieve some of the burdensome weight it necessarily brings. Surely it's psychologically easier to recover from something specific rather than an all-pervasive everything?

I am not malignant; the polyp in and around one small area of my bowel is: 21mm to be precise! Thinking ahead I'm wondering if I will have to tick the 'Have you had cancer?' box for any future medical appointments or health insurance forms. For now that box categorically remains blank. I don't want to be scarred for life with a full-blown cancer diagnosis.

Have you had a cancer diagnosis, or been given any other chronic illness label?

....

....

....

Have you given any thought to how you refer to your illness?

....

....

....

Can you think of another way to refer to your situation that empowers your body and your mind's capacity to heal?

....

....

....

14 June 2011

The Waiting Game

Agonising suspense, major denial, nervous twitches and butterflies are consuming and extending far beyond my stomach's reach; the countdown to D-day has begun.

Should I think about it? Or not? Even if I were to avoid it, would I manage? I can't control my anxious and wondering mind. I'm overwhelmed by everything I want to squeeze in beforehand: taking Rufus to the vet for his annual immunisations; stocking up on his gold-plated, new-age, sensitive-stomach dry food; getting my hair cut and my legs waxed. I've been told to strip my toenails of any polish as during anaesthesia they provide a visual indication of oxygen levels. What a lovely thought—not. Then there's the pantry, fridge and freezer to stock up. It's like my own personal preparatory Armageddon. Transferring CFO (Chief Financial Officer) duties to Danny, currently our family's CNFO, Chief Non-Financial Officer. Teaching the children new cooking skills, whilst hurriedly imparting small snippets of motherly advice to enhance their independence and buoy their self-confidence. I also need time to soak up some rays of sunshine, absorb the green blades of grass and yellow wattle blazing in the winter sunshine, cuddle the dog and of course the kids! There are just not enough hours in the day.

Who to call? Who not to call? Who to text? Who not to text? Who to email, Skype, Facebook? I'm grateful I don't have a Twitter account and LinkedIn is purely professional.

The thinking game. Everything relates to my perception of how I will be pre and post-op. And it's not just short-term; I can't refrain from future projections either.

Is it naïve to be excitedly optimistic about a future immeasurably rosier and healthier? My mood is vacillating like clouds drifting across a windswept sky. I am trying to halt negative thoughts, telling myself to put them on imaginary leaves flowing in the imaginary stream in my mind. It's what my new visualisation CD tells me to do. But my mind keeps clogging up. I can't even access a clear picture of the stream, as for the leaves … Are they autumnal or deciduous? Oh crikey, just stop! I wonder how many negative thoughts remain steadfastly clumped together and how many have escaped.

More than ever I recognise the truth in the statement: 'It takes a lot of strength to be strong!' As this episode fades into the next instalment of my life, I choose to be strong. I will be invincible. I will be so strong and mighty that, as I power down the pavement, people may point in my direction, and quietly murmur, 'Wow she might not look Schwarzenegger-esque, but you can really feel her power.'

Strength may not be something we are born with, literally or figuratively, but it is certainly something we can build, grow, nurture and work towards. It is in these challenges (big, small, and often daunting) and through all those emotional workouts and years of tests, trials and tribulations that we grow the strongest.

From mini to mighty. From pastel to bold. From dependant to independent.

Night night. xx

What experiences have made you stronger?

....

....

....

In what ways?

....

....

....

15 June 2011

The night before the night before

Tentatively we touched each other knowing that the next time we made love, things would be very different. The enormity of what lay ahead was too daunting. I buried myself in Danny's caress, but the intimacy just brought me to tears. We had to make love once more. I wanted to, but how could we in such a sombre state?

The second opinion we received provided us with a sketchily drawn illustration of the bowel resection and where it fitted into the female body, wedged right amidst reproductive organs. For men, this is an easier operation. No risk to reproductive health and functions, but as the surgeon explained, for women, in cutting and remodelling parts of the bowel, due to the vagina's close proximity (like a shared border) there was a chance they may be forever altered. At the time I didn't think this was a good enough reason not to go ahead with the operation although I had been told a similar tale prior to childbirth, that weeing may never feel the same, and it had been true in my case.

So now there was even more pressure on this final time to make love. It might not ever feel the same. It was all just too much to bear … more tears!

Like pillows stuffed with stones we lay there; our voices non-verbal, our emotions too emotional. Bolstered by our love for each other, yet crumbling at the same time, both too scared to make the first move. Two blind mice in the dark. Who knows what the next few days will bring. Why can't we bring ourselves to do this one act that we've done out of passion, out of our basic animal instincts, thousands of times before. Childhood sweethearts, never for one second predicting this as the road we would traverse.

Eventually it happened. Passion ran deep but silent. Afterwards we lay in each other's arms. I glanced over at Danny and witnessed a tear slowly sliding from his eye. Sluggishly it moved down his cheek before being splayed by his one-day growth. How many tears he had shed before, I don't know; but I was drowning just looking at this one teardrop. My gut was wrenching. Shedding imaginary tears, we fell asleep wrapped in each other's arms.

In so many ways this is easier for me. I'm the one going through this in my own body; he's powerless, a supportive bystander of the highest order. Neither he nor I have control over what may become; but we're both terrified.

Now, sitting here writing, I feel sorry he chose me to anchor his love, sorry for bringing the one I love most, so much pain, sorrow and heartache. Whilst others may have affairs, my health is the source of betrayal, stepping in to change plans, slow me down, and rob me of my spirit and energy.

I'm so sorry Danny I'm not a more robust specimen of health. I know you don't see things the way I do, nor likely feel this way, but that doesn't prevent the guilt from consuming me. That micro-millilitre solitary tear you tried so hard to conceal says more about the depth of our love than an entire ocean.

17 June 2011

D Day

My bowel has been prepped, matching my psychological state. I have never been so psyched for anything, ever, and wonder if I will ever feel so psychologically strong again. I will wrought iron beams to support me but still fear they might morph into cotton wool.

Once at the hospital, I was allocated cubicle number 8 which I took as a good sign. Recently I've been drawn to the significance of certain numbers. Number 8 matches the mathematical symbol of infinity and symbolises completeness or wholeness—two complete circles linked into one, resting in each other's curved arms, unable to differentiate which circle leans onto the other. I've heard it is associated with good luck, and I, for one, need all the luck I can get! June 17 also is an auspicious date adding up to another 8! I may be clutching at straws but if it helps, why not?

Danny was still allowed at my side. I was certain we were both feeling sick to our stomachs. Sentences were filled with mundanities as anything else just added to our emotional load. Nurses came, nurses went. Finally the anaesthetist arrived and briefed me about what lay ahead. I would be under anaesthesia for around 5 hours. He would be monitoring my every step, and soon he would return to take me into the operating theatre. I hadn't recalled being told that the operation would be so lengthy, but as long as they did a good job I doubted a lengthier operation would make any difference in the long run. I don't know how warm it really was but I was shivering out of nerves and a blood supply that had largely taken leave of absence.

The next thing I knew my legs were wrapped in lightweight

silver coils, like a 3-dimensional slinky, but nowhere near as fun. Apparently this was to assist with circulation and would be left on my legs until after the operation. From waist down I looked like an extra-terrestrial being and wished I could be beamed up right away! Next, the surgeon appeared asking me if I had any questions, but I got the impression it was cursory. I was straight-jacketed to the bed and it was way too late for any questions, even if they were perfunctory. I just wanted this to be over, to be on the other side.

I avoided looking directly into Danny's eyes as the floodgates in both him and myself weakened with each shallow breath. Time was running out. Soon they would be collecting me. A nurse by the name of Emily (another good sign—my sister's name) came to my bed and said she would be at my side the entire duration of the operation, as my surgeon played God. She didn't leave though. It was time. Enveloped in panic I turned to Danny for one last hug goodbye. We were both shaking and I sensed he was losing the battle to stay strong. A trademark of a long-distance relationship, Danny being from the UK and I from Melbourne, we'd had so many emotional farewells. Yet as heart-wrenching as they might have been, they paled in comparison. Sure there may have been the occasional infinitesimal fear of a plane crash or of an even more perfect match appearing out of nowhere and severing our love, but deep down we knew we would return to each other's embrace.

Now I was a mother. We had kids. This was an absolutely humungous operation, classified between a hysterectomy and heart surgery; but the whopping 5 hours more closely aligned with heart surgery. Like all operations it bore a risk, not only to my inner functions but also to my existence. I pushed back that torrent of thought. Nope, I was not going there. My voice strained as I uttered my final words, 'I'll see you on the other side.' I couldn't even be sure Danny heard them. Too scared to even cry, I was wheeled into the operating Temple of stainless steel, complete with bright lights, beeping and computer screens. Everyone was pleasant enough and did their best to play down the seriousness of what was to follow. An intravenous (IV) bung was inserted in my hand. 'Just a little sting,' said the anaesthetist. I beckoned all the love, support and protection I had in this world and summoned the same from other worlds. I visualised the Lion of Judah with an outstretched paw keeping any evil at bay and the love of both my beloved grandmothers now deceased. I never knew my maternal grandfather and my paternal grandfather passed when I was just a toddler, but I was sure they were there shielding me from harm's way. I was bathed in universal love. On instruction I counted slowly to ten, then my consciousness surrendered. I was in their hands.

X

Between Two Worlds: To The Other Side

I was being wheeled down a narrow corridor when my eyes opened just long enough to see a panic-stricken Danny walking beside me. Apparently I emitted a groan, and then I was out again.

I next awakened in a recovery room. My eyes were open, but I was not fully present. I felt like I was falling and falling. I couldn't make any words come out of my mouth; they were stuck. A nurse came to check on me. I have a vague recollection of her saying something about how long I took to wake up (I later found out it had been several hours and I was in intensive care). Immobilised, I still couldn't speak, sinking deeper and deeper. I was in my body, but my heart barely was. I passed through both sides of consciousness, at times feeling closer to death than life. My frantically pulsating anchor was unmooring, seemingly trying to exit its own cavity. I wanted to be back in the here and now, but was between two worlds, neither of them comforting. I couldn't breathe, nor move or motion for the nurse to remove my oxygen mask. Couldn't they see I couldn't breathe? It felt like oxygen was being syphoned away rather than supplied. Powerless, trapped and voiceless, I willed my eyes to open. I wished someone could have stayed by my side to hold my hand and comfort me. Why did they have to keep disappearing? All I could see were empty beds.

Finally my mask was removed, but still I was sinking deeper. Words once again failed me. My heart rate was over 128 beats per minute, at times faster. I faintly overheard discussions about the need to page my anaesthetist and another nurse saying it was nearly 3am. 3am? How could it be? My operation was at 2pm. Simultaneously I wanted to throw up and pass out. Thankfully I must have surrendered to sleep because when I next opened my eyes I was in a different room with 5 or so other people—one of them screaming to get the nurses' attention. The beeping of machines filled the room; that and the loud cries of the woman opposite me. Why was she so inconsiderate? Couldn't she see she was not the only one here? I needed peace and quiet. My heart still seemed to be beating extraneously from my body. I felt like death warmed up yet mustered a smile when a kindly nurse asked if I wanted an oxygen mask. No way did I want that suffocating apparel anywhere near me again. Instead I opted for more morphine.

At least I knew I was alive! I just couldn't move more than a millimetre without pain gripping every part of my body neck down.

What a mammoth operation, to put it mildly! No one could have prepared me for its enormity. And I don't blame them; how could they? Thankfully with no live experience of operations (save for wisdom teeth extraction) my only point of reference in terms of non-worldly pain was childbirth, and what a doddle that was!

Thank you from the bottom of my heart for delivering me to the other side. I am filled with boundless gratitude for all the love and support I have received. Let the healing and recovery begin!

Xoxoxoxoxoxoxo

20 June 2011

Time in Hospital

Seconds feel like minutes, minutes like hours, hours like days. Time passes agonisingly slowly. Willing it to go quicker is counterproductive; the clock ticks even slower. The hands on my watch are my enemy. A cheap Thai special, the hour hand does not fall on the hour and in the dim and darkened night light. I can never be sure of the exact time. I have been tricked into thinking it was a full hour later only to downheartedly realise on closer inspection it is a full hour earlier. Can't it be morning yet?

I am slowly becoming accustomed to a different rhythm. At home, mornings begin anytime from the first bird song to the rude awakenings of the neighbour's courier vans revving into action. Obnoxious noise pollution, together with real pollution, infiltrates and permeates our slumber and bedroom. Here I drift in and out of consciousness marred by the sounds of beeping drip machines, alarms ringing and the shuffling of nurses' footsteps bypassing my room. The closest thing to a 6.45am alarm call is the clanging of the water trolley, getting louder and louder as it approaches my bedroom door. I want it to go away. Please leave me alone.

I strain to utter 'no ice' as my raspy first words of the day, belatedly followed by a guilty 'thank you'. Every morning I wonder how people can begin their day by imbibing an icy cold fluid that jolts their inner system in a manner more akin to shock therapy than hydration therapy. Surely the best and kindest thing for your body is to drink beverages at room temperature or even warmer?

Please can't time pass quicker? Can't I be well enough to go home already? I don't know what's worse at times, the physical pain or the pain of time passing so slowly. I lie around waiting. In theory I'd love to have visitors but am in no way up to it. I'm not used to 'being visited' as a passive patient. Revealing a part of myself that should only be shared with the closest of family or friends is just not something I'm comfortable with. I'm not on exhibition.

Let's face it, I feel lousy. Yet, I am fully aware that I am the lucky one. I think of all those patients whose stays in hospitals are so long that the familiarity of home fades into something from the past—unattainable and removed—a distant memory, and perhaps one that will stay as just that.

I continue staring at the hands of my watch as they slowly tick over. On the one hand I relax into the moment and count my blessings; whilst on the other I conjure up images of my body being able to heal in fast-forward motion, like time-lapse photography.

Recount a time when time has moved agonisingly slowly.
What, if anything, did you do to speed up the passage of time? Did it help?

....
....
....
....
....
....

21 June 2011

Regrowth...Reborn

Today a lady bearing a folder and friendly disposition came into my room enquiring if I would be happy to be part of a National Colorectal Cancer Audit—a database administered by the hospital with patient information to inform best-practice and research. As a public health practitioner I did not need any convincing. Feeling useful and with a renewed sense of purpose, unhesitatingly I signed up. She stayed a few moments before leaving an information sheet for me to read.

Her footsteps petered out into the room next door as I glanced at the sheet. On it was an explanation of the operation I had just had, and would you believe it, the name for this procedure derives from the Ancient Greek word neoplasia meaning 'new growth'. Just another confirmation that perhaps—at an existential or unconscious level—I chose this procedure to allow myself to grow. Indeed, what better way to enable growth than surgery? You can't be more clear-cut than that. Out with the old!

I'm constantly amazed at the array of positive things that have occurred these past weeks. I feel so supported, and it's not just because of earthly love. Honestly I feel like a band of genies magically appeared when the rug was rudely ripped from under my feet, some grasping its four corners whilst others shuffled around supporting any sagging areas. Then rather than succumb to the harsh disorienting fall I feared, I landed on a pile of life-sized marshmallow, not slap bang and out of control. For this I am eternally grateful.

Since my decision to have the 'peace of mind' operation, I feel as though I've been given an opportunity to metamorphose, to be reborn. Reinforcing this feeling is the fact that the operation somehow rebooted my personal calendar. The day after became 'Day one post-op', followed by 'Day two post-op' akin to a baby being born. Today I am nine days old!

As with babies, after a bowel resection food is introduced gradually and slowly with notes taken on any reaction or allergy. Some assimilate and digest well, while others leave me with chronic diarrhoea, pain and bloating. There's no other way of putting it, this wind and inexplicable pain feels like colic!

Babies are loved unconditionally; everyone showers them in love—same with me. I have been bathed in so much love, which has been absolutely remarkable and extremely comforting.

I delight in minor achievements; taking my first step post-op, also lauded by staff, which in time has resulted in more adventurous ward walks that were marvelled and praised. So much love, so much encouragement.

At some level, perhaps, this shows me what it is like to be born, once again: being helpless, dependent and desirous of unconditional love and support. I've had people washing me, wiping me down and cleaning away my poo. I even have deodorised nappy sacks and a spare bag 'just in case'. Friends have cooked for my family and showered me with gifts. Even people I rarely see, but whose friendship used to feature in my life, have demonstrated their love through action or words.

It's so sad to think how many people are deprived of love and encouragement during their life course. Not just external praise but also internal praise, loving ourselves for what we really are: perfectly imperfect human beings.

I now really appreciate what it means to be in this world. I am much wiser yet recognise that, even with all the knowledge and wisdom that has been bestowed in my 43 years, I am continually being reborn, continually evolving and continually growing. I am contemplating how little I know and how much there is to learn in this gift that we refer to as life.

X

Has there been a time in your life when you felt helpless and dependent on others?

....

....

....

Who helped you through this time?

....

....

....

Have you ever let them know how much this meant to you?

....

....

....

Why not send them a letter or email, or even pick up the phone and say thanks.

Card from Rufus

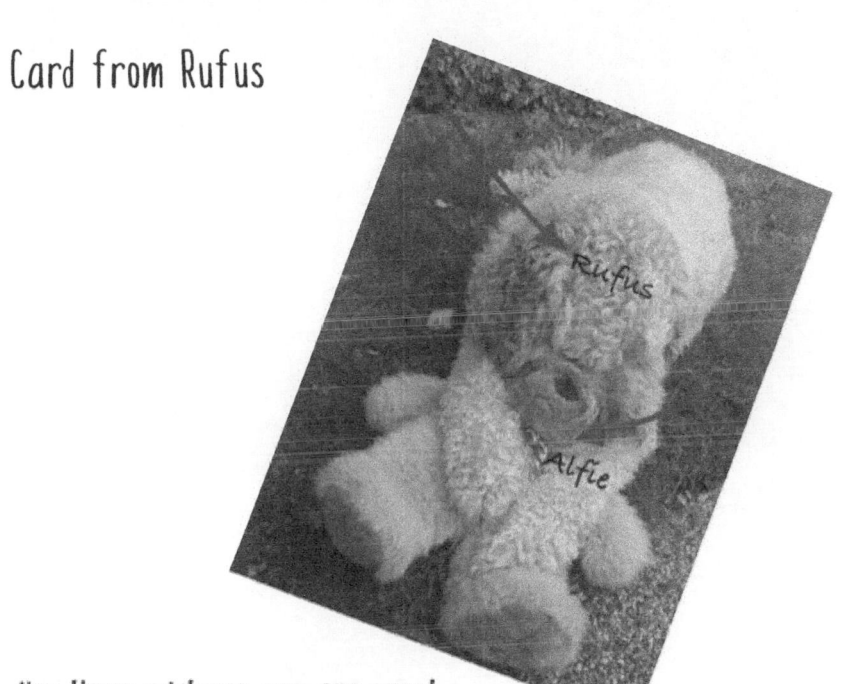

Hey there mistress, you are great
This is _me_ dreaming about our next date

I think you have gone on a trip
To bring me back chicken necks quick

Life's so great when I see you
I love snuggling in that's what I do

I want you to know the park is waiting for you
I'm sure you are desperate to take me there as you often
do

By the time you come home my fur will be long
And if you need someone fat to lean on then I am sure
strong

Lots of love mistress, I mean dear goddess
And regards from *Alfie whose hair is a mess

(*Alfie is Rufus's bear that he takes wherever he goes and has
done since he was a puppy.)

22 June 2011

Changing bags

'I have always been fond of my bottom' might be a funny line to begin a journal entry, but is true nonetheless.

When I was told my rectum would be removed, I immediately envisaged my bottom would somehow assume a different shape or form, but of course it was only an internal modification.

Prior to surgery I had an appointment with a stomal therapy nurse who briefed me on what to expect. Despite having worked in health promotion for many years, I had never heard of a stomal therapist, and neither had spell-checks, judging by the persistent red line appearing underneath the word as I type it. Most matter-of-factly I was told I would be fitted with a bag that would sit on the outside of my stomach. Moreover a loop from my bowel would extend beyond the confines of my neatly packaged and cute abdomen (OK, I added that last bit), which would empty directly into the attached bag. She had even added, cheekily, 'The surgeon will love you, you're so slim. It will make his work so much easier.' Who would have thought my slim build could be so advantageous in moments like these.

Trying to get my head around the enormities of my surgery, knowingly or otherwise, I blocked out any thoughts of this alien concept. It was just not something I had the energy or headspace to deal with. If ever I did start to think about it, my thoughts automatically shifted to very old people in residential aged care. This was the demographic for which I had heard references about 'bags' and in my mind, somehow, it seemed more normal and acceptable in this age group. Within the scheme of things, this really seemed like the least of my worries.

During my gradual reawakening from the operation, I sensed the presence of a bag resting on my skin, but in my all-consuming excruciating pain not even momentarily did I consider lifting my gown to inspect.

The shock came two days thereafter. And when I say shock, I mean horror, terror and other related synonyms. The stomal therapist, Helen, in the nicest of ways reminds me of the blue healer five doors down, 100% true blue Aussie. My patchwork stomach, ever so tender from surgical incisions, was ill-prepared for what was to come: excruciating, searing pain as the adhesive seal of the bag was delicately peeled off. Picture Brazilian waxing a gorilla and you may come close to imagine the sensation I felt as every microscopic hair was yanked one by one.

Gazing down I was gripped by horror as a penile looking extrusion extending from my stomach stared back at me. I blinked and blinked again, but my eyes did not deceive me. I had woken up with a phallus sticking out of my body! I wonder if males find it easier bonding with their stomas?

My brain, still in shock, was trying to process this when my olfactory system kicked in and a vile and putrid smell wafted into my nostrils. Never before had I encountered such a smell. If it had a colour it would be a thick cloud of mustard yellow/green, and a visual would be the cartoon skunk, Pepe Le Pew.

I had been forewarned, but it's like preparing a blind person for sight, or a deaf person for sound. I felt woozy from the sight of this penis extruding from my stomach sickened by the stench and wounded by the pain not only emanating from every muscle and cell within my body, but from the recently ripped adhesive that firmly bound the bag to my flesh.

Thankfully, in my pained and weakened state, all I had to do was lie where I was, and Helen did the rest. 'So how many times does this bag need to be changed?' I whispered in trepidation. 'Every two days,' was certainly not the response I had hoped to hear. Presumably, unless I stayed in hospital (God forbid) for the next 3 months, this meant I bore sole responsibility for changing it. God give me strength!

In the back of my mind, I began questioning the need for this operation—after all, it had been optional. What had I got myself into here? I could have chosen the lesser op and avoided this bag. But Ian Gawler's words, 'Make a decision and enjoy it; don't look back,' quickly steered my mind away from irrelevant and damaging retrospections. The stoma will optimise healing around my bowel and rectum. As explained by the surgeon, in this nether region, blood supply and therefore healing is slower than other body parts. Yes Ros, this stoma is for your own good! OK, back on track.

Four days post-op, Helen returned to my hospital room with an air of excitement. 'OK, your turn,' she announced. Already? Really? Moreover, instead of changing it lying down, she told me it was best to change it in the bathroom, followed by a shower.

On the assumption that the bathroom and shower wouldn't come to me, this meant I needed to get to them. 'I can do it!' streamed through my consciousness, somehow propelling me out of bed to shuffle the ten or so agonising steps to the bathroom. 'I can do it. I can do it,' the internal voice in my head kept repeating. I am young; I am a health professional, and this is just how it has to be. And then the mantra from The Little Engine That Could, 'I think I can,' pulling the train over the mountain striving for the top of the hill, allowed me to transport from bed to bathroom, buoyed by Helen at my side.

All essential equipment was laid out on the sink: the new bag (baby bags were so much more interesting), two chux wipes, a disposable scented bag and some toilet paper. It was as if I was a new mum, learning to change my baby's first nappy.

Filled with intense angst, I summoned great resolve and braced myself for the task ahead. Looking at all the paraphernalia laid out around the sink, this process felt as removed from second nature as could be.

OK, some deep breaths. Well theoretical deep breaths, as my insides felt like they would rip, explode and splat in multiple directions with the shallowest of breaths.

'I can do it, I can do it,' piped my inner engine as I slowly peeled the adhesive away from my skin. I was doing it! Wipes at bay, I tentatively wiped the areas with a pre-dampened wipe and then even more tentatively dried it with the other wipe. 'Don't be afraid,' Helen offered. 'Give it a real wipe, then dry it thoroughly.'

Then my olfactory system kicked in and whatever colour had been in my face instantly drained away. Thankfully, the ever-dependable Helen was quick at her feet and steered the nearby plastic chair in my direction, catching me as I semi fainted into it.

How many weeks to go?

When Things don't go to plan

Today is the day I was meant to be discharged. Last night I had gone to bed soaring with the wonderful news we had all been waiting to hear, that the cancer had not spread. But in the wee evening hours I was alerted to a weird sensation as a bloody stench discharged from my anus streaming out onto my sheet. How could this be? This area had been sealed off? I reached for the call button at lightning bolt speed and waited many long moments before a nurse came to my side. By then, I was a quivering wreck consumed with thoughts of death and emergency surgery.

Seeing the state I was in, the nurse immediately called for backup. They lost no time, investigating what was going on and unhesitatingly reassured me it was old discharge and all was OK. Apparently this sometimes happened, but they reiterated that the bowel had definitely been sealed and that no new waste could or would travel out of my anus. They left me to try and fall back to sleep, but my mind was on fire, and I was still very much in a state of shock.

Somehow, time passed and daylight peeped through the curtain. I was in a bad way, still shaken and upset that no one had warned me this could happen. My thoughts went to the girls who, left uninformed on the topic of their period, are immobilised by shock and fear as blood streams down the inside of their legs.

The last thing I felt like was eating the breakfast that had just been delivered. I felt as dark as the night sky recently departed and in no mood to eat. I wanted to mope and was feeling exceedingly sorry for myself. This was meant to be discharge day, and this was certainly not the discharge I had in mind.

Staring me in the eyes was a large white hospital placemat lining the untouched meals tray. It beckoned me. Clearing some space, I mapped out a tiny, thin column and began writing. I started listing everything I was grateful for in my current situation, such as appreciating how miraculous every functioning part of the body is; the importance of slowing down, even if it had been enforced; and the body's miraculous capacity to heal. I glanced at the large void on the remaining space and felt compelled to continue writing.

Quite unexpectedly, I was consumed by feelings of profound gratitude and deep love for myself, others and just being alive. A beaming smile now replaced the look of sheer terror that had gripped me moments before. Not only was I smiling, but, just by focusing on these wondrous life-affirming feelings, I became aware my whole body was smiling. It was as if every cell, every tissue and every aching muscle was filled with the love embodied in this genuine, heart-felt smile. Inwardly I laughed (laughing outwardly would have led to searing pain) as my writing got smaller and more cramped, and I struggled to squeeze everything I wanted to say into the diminishing space.

I had done it. From bleakness came light. From fear came love, and with it, an inner conviction that it would only be a matter of time before I was laughing and really living again, surrounded by my loved ones. When the same nurse who had comforted me earlier came to check in on me, to her surprise and delight, I greeted her with a smile.

I finally made peace with a warrior of a day. It has shown me that even in the face of seeming adversity there exists the potential to find positive things. I still can't believe they leaped off the page!

I'm recalling how early into my journey one of my dearest friends Dani, recounted something said to her after she had relayed my shock diagnosis, 'You only see stars in a darkened sky'. And today I can honestly say I have seen them shine.

All being well tomorrow will be my homecoming, blessed by good health, happiness and lots of love. What a journey. What an experience. What a STORY!

X X X X X X X X

Have you ever tried reframing painful situations through writing? Take some time now to think of a time that was particularly painful or challenging. List as many positives as you can relating to that situation. Acknowledging even the smallest positive outcome can help shift pain.

....
....
....
....
....
....
....
....

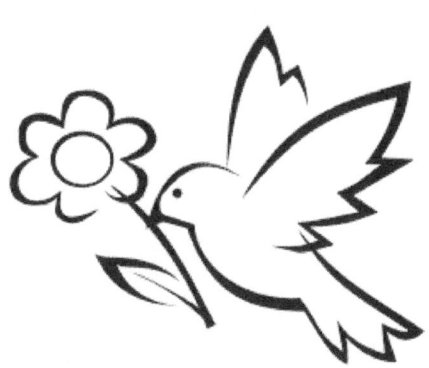

All the Positives

- Get into the habit of eating slower and really chewing food
- Slow down generally
- Appreciate how miraculous every functioning part of my body is
- Appreciate the body's capacity to heal
- To learn healing techniques
- Learn/adopt/habituate meditation
- Enjoy gazing out from my hospital window the beautiful Dandenong Ranges in the horizon
- Appreciate nature and its positive effect on my wellbeing
- Having this operation in a world-class hospital
- Really appreciate being alive
- To find the positives even when things seem grim, such as anal discharge
- Know that it's much better to be rid of the old
- Feel how much love is out in the world — really "feel the love"
- Gain understanding of my weaknesses and strengths
- Test bravery
- Have faith
- Trust in my body's innate wisdom and its amazing ability to heal - truly miraculous!
- Time to just "be"
- Time out to reconfigure, reinvent, reprioritise and restructure
- Make real life resolutions
- Know my anal passage is still intact
- Appreciate all the wonderful things & people in my life — children, Danny, extended family and extraordinary friends
- Appreciation of the attentive hospital staff (cleaners, doctors, nurses and room service attendants)
- Amazement of number of smiles from everyone here, bottom up
- Gain new wisdom
- How many positives I have come up with without having to think too much
- Relaxation, even when the environment may not be naturally conducive
- Not panic (still working on that!)
- WOW! How blessed am I!!

Saturday 25 June 2011

Homecoming

Wow! What better way to mark this momentous occasion than to initiate and induct this special pen for this journal entry. Carved from recycled wood from an old Victorian country bridge that dates back to 1880, it was lovingly given to me by my sister-in-law, Dalia, in the days leading up to my operation.

I woke up to Day 8 post-op after a comfortable night's sleep. The body is such a miraculous machine. What it has achieved in the past eight days is akin to a whole city bulldozed to its core, rising up once again. Thank God for all the wonderful healing energy and universal love I have received to reach this special day.

The nurse drew back the curtains to reveal a clear blue sky. As my eyes transitioned from night to day, I saw the Dandenong Mountain ranges in the distance, and slowly, one of three hovering hot air balloons drifted into view against the backdrop of the perfectly blue sky. What a sight! What a spectacular blessing of a day to be alive! Thank you.

I took a moment to consider some of the amazing things that have typified this life-affirming experience: people's extraordinary capacity for good, to be kind, loving and generous of heart.

With a magnificent red rose clamped between his large pearl-white teeth, Danny arrived promptly at 10.15am (a miracle in itself for anyone familiar with Danny's idea of time-keeping) to deliver me to my rightful place: home. I couldn't quite believe I could even dare to utter that sentence, 'I really am on my way home!'

In moments like these I am filled with deep gratitude and profound love for Danny, too often taken for granted in day-today living. I see specks of gold in this lifetime pile of silt, rising to the surface, glistening and glowing in full splendour.

Discharge form in hand, wearing clothes for the first time in eight days, I transformed almost seamlessly from patient to person in only a few moments, and boy did it feel great.

Despite my uncertain, weak steps, I enthusiastically made my way out of the ward, saying goodbye to the familiar faces who had been my salvation for the past eight days. The amazing staff who had excelled in making me as comfortable and cared for as humanly possible.

Now, after eight days of being indoors, in an artificially controlled environment, I stepped into a fresh, new day. People were getting on with whatever they were doing: walking, working, hopping on and off trams, crossing the lights, shopping and so on. To them, it was just another ordinary day blending into the tally of days that pass without anything special happening.

Yet, I was bedazzled, totally in awe, and had to pause a moment to breathe in the fresh, crisp air, as deeply as my pained insides would allow. So good! I just had to ingest some more and savour this sweetness, this elixir of life. To savour what so many people, myself included, take for granted; at first, breathing unconsciously before consciously inhaling this revitalising, pure, unadulterated air. Nothing fabricated, or manufactured there—minus daily pollutants such as car fumes—just the natural balance of oxygen in and carbon dioxide out: an invisible life force.

Danny pointed in the direction of the car, saying, 'It's just over there, past the traffic lights.' I calculated how many rounds of hospital ward corridors his 'over there' amounted to. It was quite a distance, but who cared, I was free! Free in a literal and physical sense. What an absolutely liberating, awesome sensation. This time last week I couldn't move one centimetre without wincing in crippling pain, and now, just one week and one day later, I was slowly and ever so gingerly walking down a busy road to our car! Once again, I needed to pause in wondrous reflection at the awesome capacity of our bodies to heal, regenerate and rebuild. Truly remarkable!

Then, without even too much effort, I was in the car, and

we were on our way. It was surreal, like an eternity had passed since I was in the real world. The sky was a brilliant blue; the trees gently swayed as we zoomed past picture-perfect houses and manicured gardens. I marvelled at the seemingly unremarkable, yet in my present state of mind, the ever so remarkable. My internal dimmer switch was at its brightest setting.

En route we made a short stop at the green grocer to satiate my desire to eat sweet potato (one of the few vegetables I can actually digest), and I remained in the car contemplating the enormity of the past week's events. I drew down the passenger mirror to see a face somewhat thinner, slightly paler, with a new growth of eyebrow stubble, yet remarkably intact. I don't know what I was expecting to see, but cautiously I exhaled in mild relief. With my fingers, I began gently reshaping my eyebrows in an attempt to feel a little more outwardly groomed when I was alerted to a tap on my window as the door handle gently pulled open. Our family's long standing barber had interrupted a client's haircut to give me a kiss, wish me well and tell me how he looked forward to seeing me shopping in suburban Carnegie 'in no time at all'. He farewelled me with an enthusiastic and warm 'ciao', instantly filling my face with colour. How very special!

Finally we pulled into our drive. I gently manoeuvred the clasp of the seat belt and with a hint of trepidation sashayed out of the car, journeying to the front door propelled by willpower alone. I could not believe I was back on home turf, when just a short while prior I had been a patient lying in a hospital bed with my heart and blood pressure monitored.

The silhouettes of Zak, Josh and Rufus lined the inside of the doorway, and they quickly descended, cued by a series of hoots. I was immediately lovingly showered with hugs and kisses accompanied by visibly immense relief at seeing mum finally home. As for Rufus, if his body could have merged into mine in his embrace, it would have, and although his rather large build and shaggy fur made me slightly anxious as he snuggled in, I felt no discomfort, just gentle, tender love. His love was weightless, unlike his BMI, not too dissimilar to mine following these gruelling weeks.

Straight away I was presented with magnificent, individually designed cards which I paused to admire before shuffling a little further forward to the piece de resistance: a floral path composed of deep-red rose petals leading into our home. It was beyond words. To return to this glorious sight infused by love, romance and beauty almost in itself merited the past week of pain and longing. I needed nothing else. Everything was contained within these walls: my home, filled with the treasures of my (our) creation: my family!

Oh, to savour this perfect moment. The sun streamed in through the living room windows, loving, excited children and doting husband at my side. All of us in our own way delighting in my homecoming. Back home where I belonged. Lunch was a simple affair but could not have been more perfect. Eating with my family, my children; something I have taken for granted, even mildly dreaded at times, yet now am soaking in every little bit of, drenched by their looks of joy, impeccable behaviour, and the occasional sidling up of a cuddly and adorable pooch.

To think these things are often referred to as the 'simple things' in life; yet 'simple' does not seem to be an apt description. Surely these are the most complex? After all, they are formed by years of combining physical and emotional experiences—the entangling of lives. The simple life, that of a nuclear family, is probably one of the most complex interrelationships in existence and possibly the single most amazing miracle that ever was. A combination of each and every individual life—each a miracle in its own right— meeting your life soul mate (if you are indeed blessed to have done so), and producing more human beings sparked by miraculous beginnings. This is an example of the deficiencies of the English language and a disservice to the true meaning of 'a simple life'.

I am making a mental note to savour this feeling, so when mundane routine and sameness begins sneaking in, I can rekindle it to saturate each and every cell in my body. How extraordinarily lucky I am to have who I have in my life. 'It only takes one seed to grow a tree.'

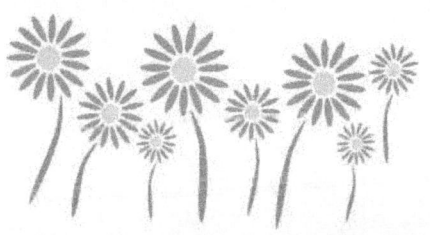

What memory or experience can you recall that you would really like to savour?

....
....
....

Write it down and put it in a place visible for your eyes only, so you can refer to it in moments of need.

....
....
....

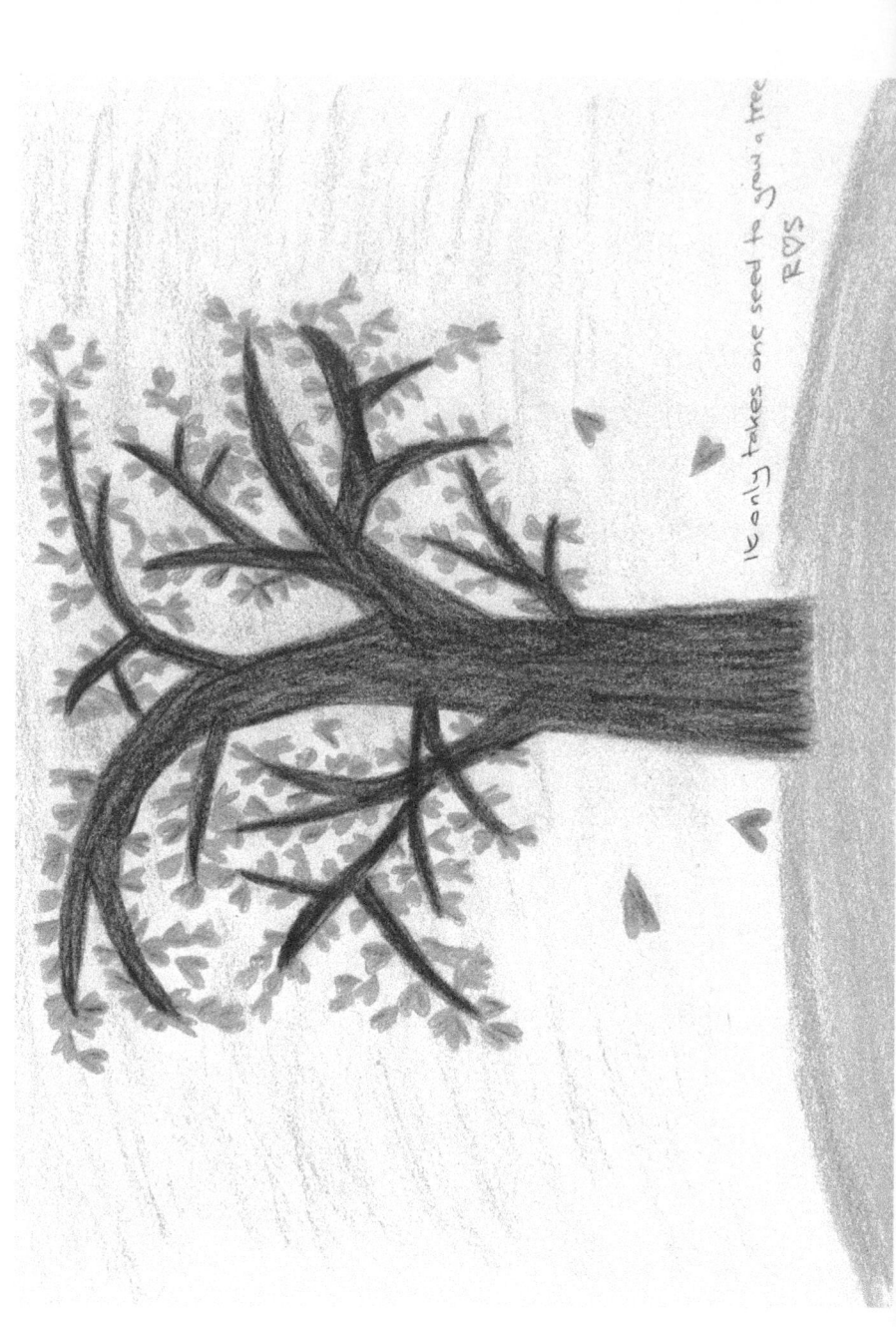

It only takes one seed to grow a tree
RVS

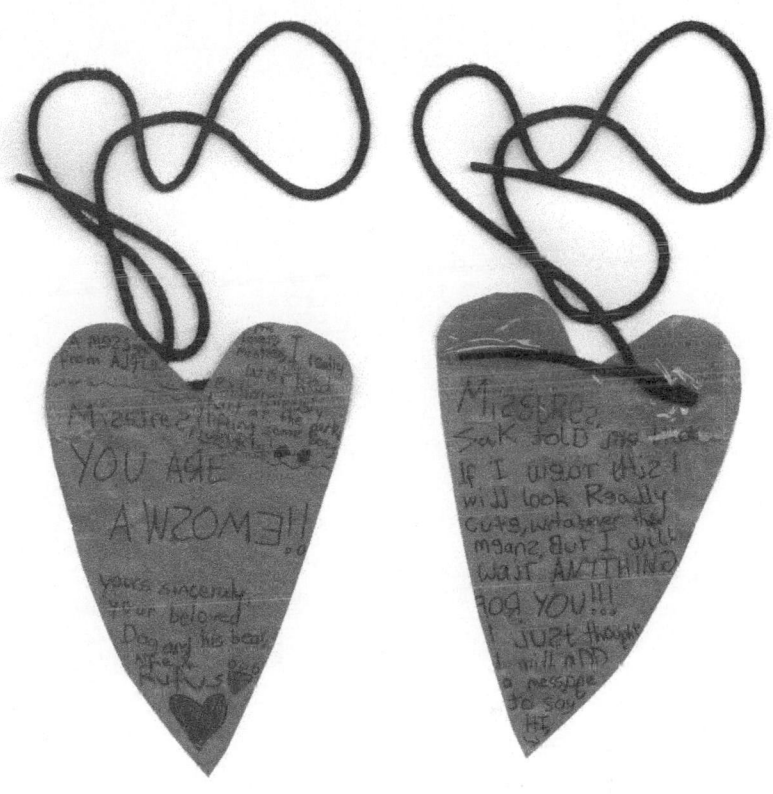

(Above: Welcome back home message from Rufus
[Dog whispering courtesy of Zak])

30 June 2011

Active Mind, not so active body

The bright light of my mind switches on, and despite my attempts to dim it, at what seems like an ungodly hour, it's no use. If only there was a physical lever I could grab hold of to dim my thoughts, induce sleep, or at least open the door to sleepy waves of relaxation. But no, my mind won't shut up. If the thoughts generated were pithy, ground breaking or revolutionary that would be one thing, but they are totally inane, inconsequential and unmatched to these wee hours. Even conjuring up imaginary streams whisking thoughts away on imaginary leaves takes me to a further barrage of thoughts, sinking any remnants of floating leaves.

I need to train my mind to switch off. Yet the harder I try, the harder it is, especially in these quiet, still and darkened hours. A screeching cat possibly on heat and the odd car accelerating down the street blend with the enviable deep-breathing sounds exuded by my sleeping husband.

So close to sleep on so many occasions, before my mind rudely stirs me with more inane, uninvited thoughts. Finally my body, mind and soul submit to sleep. Peace at last, but then the alarm calls in the guise of a child needing to be taken to school. Uggh … oh well, at least it works; the mind that is!

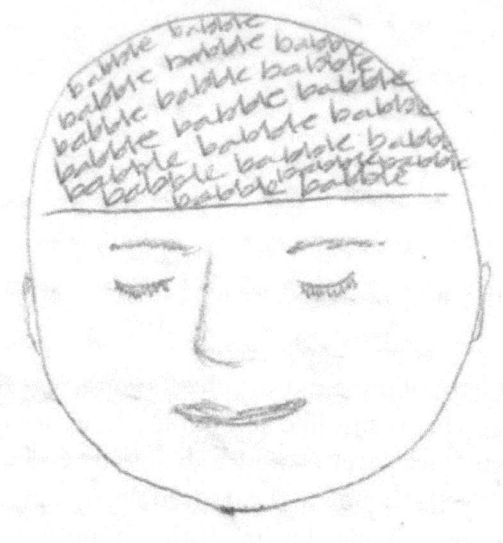

What do you do when you can't sleep?

....

....

. ...

If a barrage of thoughts plagues you in the wee hours, it's a great idea to keep a notepad by your bedside to soak some of these up.

3 July 2011
The laughter's back!

As a consequence of surgery, particularly in the abdominal area, my mobility is severely hindered, to put it mildly! Every millimetre of movement brings with it searing pain, unlike anything I have previously experienced, and yes I have given birth naturally twice!

With each passing day and the grateful assistance of some seriously strong drugs—synthetic morphine—the simple act of breathing, turning onto another side and even sitting up, gradually and for short spurts of time is becoming more bearable. The first step post-surgery was like standing on an electric cable, sending flinching, searing pain to parts of my body that usually lie dormant and still. I prayed I wouldn't catch a virus as passing nurses, visitors and other patients coughed carelessly, sending their germs flying and fragmenting in the air faster than the speed of sound.

Now I pray I won't sneeze but not as much as I pray I won't succumb to a bout of the giggles or laughter. No, that would be just too painful. I have already banned one friend from visiting, as she is a walking liability with her delightfully hearty and infectious laugh. Usually this would be one infection that, in my laughter sessions, I'd jestingly recommend people to catch; but not me, not now. No way!

My mobility is increasing as the days pass and I have more energy for evening TV viewing. Staple family viewing tends to be comedy: Modern Family, The IT Crowd, My Family, Seinfeld, posing a distinct dilemma to my innards. It is far too premature to risk comedy.

Day 13 post surgery, Zak begs, 'Can we please watch The Young Ones?' a British comedy classic. Without even thinking about it,

I say 'sure', and then it happens. I let out a small and tentative laugh. It feels incredibly good! Before I know it, I am laughing more freely and more often. How liberating. How exhilarating, how absolutely wonderful.

I welcome laughter back into my life. Boy have I missed it! I missed the physical, mechanical nature of laughing, the post laughter buzz, the unifying qualities and the liberating feel as each laugh lightens my internal load. Welcome back laughter!

X

What do you do to help trigger laughter? Do you put on a comedy show, or get together with a good friend when the laughter just flows?

....
....
....

Your laughing self

Draw a picture of yourself laughing (it can even be on a sticky note). Then place it somewhere you can easily refer to when you need a laughter boost. You can even store it inside your wallet!

8 July 2011
Laughter really is the best medicine!

My wonderful friend Sarah, imbued with a larger than-life personality, called this morning to ask a medical question. My first thought was that one of her children was unwell as occasionally she seeks my advice as a 'seasoned' mother. Her question, delivered in a serious tone, was of quite a different nature. She wanted to know whether my ileostomy bag could split if I laughed too much. Laughing my response back to her, I told her I did not think so. Excited by this revelation, she implored me to see a film she had just viewed; another gentle nudge to activate and actualise my 'laughter as best medicine' theory.

A trip to the oncology psychologist provided me with another reminder. She suggested incorporating laughter therapy, happiness philosophies and strategies into my own recovery. Hold on a second. I thought I was supposed to be the expert on all things laughter! In the process of preaching to others I seemed to have partially neglected it in my own recovery. Perhaps I needed to be told what I already knew. Perhaps I had fallen into victim mode feeling a little helpless?

She told me to close my eyes and picture the word happiness. 'Open yourself up to the meaning of happiness and then physically embody this,' she added.

Automatically I threw back both my arms towards the ceiling with a huge smile across my face and simply and emphatically said, 'YES!'

'Fantastic,' she said. 'Do this once or twice a day.'

How simple was this? I just love it. The mere thought of doing this exercise now brings a smile to my face and infuses warm feelings of wellbeing throughout my whole being. It gets me thinking about the many ways I suggest to my clients to incorporate laughter in their daily life. It's so much easier generating laughter when shared and in good company, much more natural and effortless. Laughing alone can feel a little weird, like one-hand clapping.

Hold on a second! Listen to yourself, Ros. Even if it's challenging, just choose a method: laughter meditation or laughing at yourself in the mirror. Just do it! Practice what you preach! If you feel more comfortable doing laughter meditation, great! For the next 10-15 minutes close your eyes, relax, breathe and then smile into your whole body, building up to a laughter crescendo.

How are your clients' lives any different to yours? Don't procrastinate; don't place obstacles in the way. There's no need to feel uncomfortable. Laughter is not designed to be a minimum-of-two-participants act. That's just another example of societal conditioning, no different to the notion of eating three square meals a day, breakfast, lunch and dinner, at set intervals of the day.

Thanks, little voice in my head. I hear you. I need to spend some time altering my beliefs. I need to feel OK laughing by myself. With hesitation creeping into the last word of that sentence, I feel the need to seal this with an affirmation:

> *I am OK about laughing by myself, for myself*
> *I am OK about laughing by myself, for myself*
> *I am OK about laughing by myself, for myself!*

I will clap whilst simultaneously chanting 'ho ho, ha ha ha' to increase energy levels and manufacture laughter. First thing in the morning I'll smile and share a little giggle with myself in the bathroom mirror. I will laugh in the car and out loud while watching a funny film or TV show. I'm going to amplify my laughing self; there's no point in it remaining silent. I will incorporate a smile and laughter meditation into my current meditation practice. I will laugh for no other reason than to feel great. I will try not to feel self-conscious. I will embrace laughter wholeheartedly. If I can't do this myself, how can I expect others to? I understand that one of the reasons people hold back from laughing alone, or for no apparent reason, is because of a deep-seated fear they may be viewed as crazy. Without realising it, I too have been feeding into this notion.

I will challenge this. Surely people have done and continue to do significantly more outrageous stuff than laughing alone without judgments being made about their mental health? Getting blind drunk is one example that immediately springs to mind, and there are enough people who do that! Ironically, in a drunken stupor, people let their hair down and free themselves of any inhibitions. They laugh a lot, truly, madly and deeply! There's that mad theme coming back!

I will endeavour to laugh truly and deeply without the means of alcohol or any other stimulant. I will explain to others who may hear my singular laughter that I am laughing my way back to good health; that it's something natural, and they too should seek to activate it.

We cry by ourselves and indulge in so many other emotional and physical states solo. We need to recondition our belief systems to empower ourselves to laugh alone and for our own sake. As I write this, I am becoming curiously aware that it might be me who still needs convincing.

I imagine my family at home in earshot of my shrieks of laughter. Would I feel free of inhibition? No doubt I would feel a little uncomfortable and, as a result, would probably opt to laugh when they were not around. This is of slight concern as they are my family.

Some more work is needed, I think. Not only do I need to challenge my own beliefs system, I need to have a laughter conversation with my family to gauge their beliefs about laughing alone, being a solo laugher.

> **I am OK about laughing by myself, for myself**
> **I am OK about laughing by myself, for myself**
> **I am OK about laughing by myself, for myself**

Do you find it easy to laugh alone?

....
....
....

Do you ever laugh at, or by yourself?

....
....
....

What affirmation can you think of to bring more laughter into your life?

....
....
....

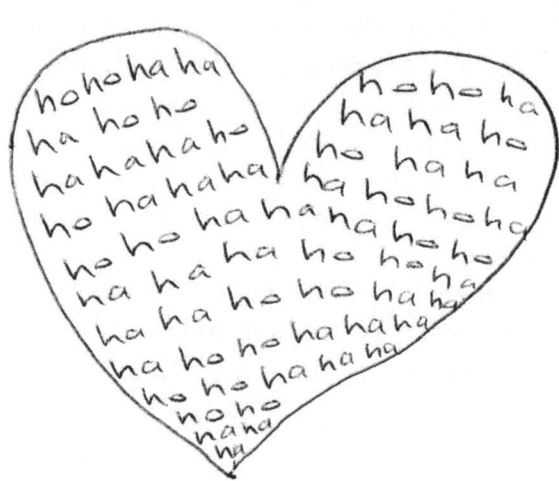

Smiling Meditation (10-15min practice)

- Make yourself comfortable sitting or lying down, and then close your eyes.
- Take some deep breaths in and out, breathing in for a count of 3, holding for 3, and then exhaling for 4. Do until you are feeling more relaxed.
- Imagine a gentle wave of relaxation—it might have a shape or colour—then allow it to gently pass throughout your whole body, beginning at the top of your head and going right down to your toes.
- Then place a genuine heartfelt smile on your face. It might help to think of a time you felt unconditionally loved, or a particular moment that filled you with love.
- Breathe the smile in and exhale it throughout your whole body until you feel every cell, every muscle, every tissue, every fibre, smiling back at you.
- How does your face feel? How do your eyes, your mouth and your whole body feel with this beautiful glowing smile?
- Know that at any time of day you can rekindle this feeling just by placing a smile on your face; a smile changes your whole physiology!

Add some laughter to this meditation practice

- Now take some more deep breaths in and out, and then begin to laugh. It might help to think of something that is funny and makes you laugh, or begin with a simulated laughter exercise (refer to www.laughlife. com.au for examples of laughter exercises).
- Just laugh for laughter's sake. Try doing this for a minute or two or even longer.
- Remember to breathe and replenish your oxygen levels.
- When you're ready open your eyes. Do you feel any different?

12 July 2011
Theory of Relativity

Danny sustained a work injury the other day. He's not usually one to complain, but he has not stopped wallowing. Prior to eating, preparing food, getting dressed, walking the dog ... you name it, he wallows in his injury. Meanwhile, I am three weeks post bowel resection, and I don't even think I'm exaggerating when I say I haven't gone on as much; in fact I've made a conscious effort to downplay the severity of my pain and discomfort, especially in the presence of the kids.

You are no doubt thinking this injury must be pretty serious, and I'm being cruel mocking him in his current state. So this is an opportunity to let your imagination run wild, to ponder just for a minute what line of work could result in this pronounced injury? Factory worker, landscape designer, perhaps an athlete? No, no, no ... not even close. Like the final line delivered in a trilogy of responses from Get Smart, the answer is, 'Would you believe a documentary filmmaker and academic?'

Drum roll please ...

His injury is ... a PAPER CUT!

It gets me thinking about how relativity affects the way we respond to the world we live in. To him, this is a gaping wound interfering with his every step (hard to believe I know) as I sit in quiet bemusement, conscious not to laugh out loud at his discomfort, fearing it may ignite internal pain.

My other ponderings on relatively relate to the passage of time. Well-intentioned friends have enquired how long ago my op was. When I tell them 'nearly one month', each and every one of them remarks, 'Wow, that's gone quickly.' My look must say it all as, hastily, my more responsive friends add, 'For us that is.' To be honest though I can't quite determine whether it feels like a short or a long period of time myself. Days have blurred into weeks with progress slow but on the whole steady.

Recalling how I was post-op, or in hospital or the week of my homecoming seems like such a long time ago. I feel like I'm a different person physically and emotionally, yet four weeks is a comparatively short time. It's one menstrual cycle, one calendar month, four Sundays, four Mondays.

I don't know exactly what to expect. Perhaps I wish for the time to come when I won't be able to recount how many weeks have passed since that momentous day. Like reverse wishing birthdays, I won't know whether it has been nine weeks, 18 weeks or even 13 months because I will have fully recovered. Although even this early into my recovery I do have an inkling I will never forget June 17th.

So now to my newest mantra: 'My life is filled with health, happiness, peace, love, laughter and brachot (Hebrew word for blessings).'

I wonder whether I've packed too much into that one, but it just feels right.

Who could ask for more? In fact, I cannot conceive of being able to be any more grateful for what I have. A life filled with great health, happiness, peace, love, laughter and brachot.

xxx

At this moment in time what mantra best suits your heart's desire? Write it down.

....

....

....

17 July 2011

Leaving Home

For several years my private (and not so private) fantasy has been to escape the household with all its menial duties and have a break — go to a retreat, chill with girl friends, basically have some time out.

A number of excuses, real and not so real, have got in the way. I'll recount some of the really good reasons:

- Money (well there never seems to be enough of that, so a little additional debt would not make too much difference)
- Schlepping (ferrying of children) issues
- Emotional void I would create by not being there 'just in case'

I am actually stopping myself right here. These seem so extraordinarily insignificant. Surely there must have been more substantive reasons? But I am drawing a blank. I really can't think of anything. Why then have I been so slow and reticent in doing what I really wanted to do? It's not like I was talking about leaving home for a month, but even that doesn't sound sooo bad.

The kids are older and have been older for a while now. Would it really matter if their routine were altered? Would it really matter if Danny was in charge of food and they had his UK special, jacket potatoes with tuna and cheese, once or even God forbid twice a week? Perhaps with some practice and instruction, Danny could add to his three-dish menu, and I don't mean a three-course meal but the total number of dishes he can cook! As a result of my foray into hospital he has proven that, with only a little bit of prompting regarding settings, even operating a washing machine does not require a PhD (if it did he could have been operating one for years). Just writing this I'm horrified in thinking perhaps Danny and I are time-travellers from the 1950s, where I'm a housewife under the façade of an educated, liberally minded, modern woman, and Danny is actually a Don Draper equivalent (without the wandering eye) under the guise of a progressive academic and filmmaker.

Perhaps I viewed going away as a luxury, or even an indulgence. Oh no, how terribly selfish that would be! Or maybe part of me felt I needed to be around because that's what we had all grown accustomed to. How would they cope? Then it dawns on me. How would I cope? No appendages, no responsibilities, like a ship without a rudder.

Danny spends weeks amounting to months travelling, pursuing his dreams making documentaries, whilst I remain dreaming of time out, quality time together and a more equitable division of household duties. The same thoughts go through my mind each time he goes away: *Maybe when he gets back I'll go away for a few days. But guess what?* Nothing happens.

First I deal with his hurt, 'Don't you want to go away with me?' Well yes, but not necessarily, I just want to go away! Then life gets in the way and time out stays a concept rather than the reality I desire, which is a shame as quality recharge-time would have gone a long way in the emotionally laden years of 2009–11. Wow, what a couple of years! Let's review:

• We moved back home after a year in the UK; moves and all they entail are inevitably unsettling

• Danny made several overseas filmmaking trips amounting to around three months. During each trip Zak got sick with some sort of bug

• Assorted viruses took host in my system, depleting my energy stores and resilience including shingles; definitely not something I would recommend

• Mum had a heart attack, but because it was a more rare muscular as opposed to vascular attack, generally considered to be less severe, I somehow convinced myself it was not that big a deal. Hello denial!

• A close relative's sudden illness

- I carried a loved one's secret around like a large sack of potatoes on my already heaving chest
- I began a new role as university lecturer and tutor with very little formal experience
- Plus the regular humdrum often referred to as 'life' or 'living'

Stress? Stress? Stress? It doesn't take a genius to figure out that a retreat, or time out was far from being self-indulgent. It was an absolute necessity. A preventative means to apportion balance and calm in my life, some inner peace and time to receive. No wonder a benign polyp lodged in my rectum and morphed into a malignant one. Work life balance, what a novel concept!

Why did I not just go ahead and do it? Why did I think I needed permission? Who controls me? Or as Zak used to say, 'Who's the boss of me?' What kind of string puppet am I? Delving deeper I recognise going somewhere by myself, for myself, scares the hell out of me, like being singularly stranded on an island. Danny has always said I'm like a pack animal. I enjoy company. It's my own company I struggle with.

Inadvertently my eight days away were spent at ~~Hospital~~ Hotel Cabrini. That could have been an eight-night retreat, or four weekends away, or two separate trips … in summation, blissful time out! And guess what? Even under those circumstances, everyone coped. Not only did they cope in a physical sense with clothes washed in time—well, at least from what I hear—but they also coped with one of the most emotionally stressful times that we, as individuals and a collective family unit, have ever gone through. Even the dog coped! I now know I have to cut those apron strings and listen to my inner voice. Everybody will cope perfectly fine, as will I.

So what conclusions can I draw? I am not as indispensable as I think. Especially because I love to give, I need time out for self-nurturing. My ability to receive has been thwarted because I tend to focus on giving too much. Moreover if I do not give to myself, I cannot expect anyone else to do so on my behalf. It is my duty to refuel myself.

From now on, I promise to go away if I feel the need. I don't necessarily have to schedule it, but I must hone into my inner voice and act upon it when the need presents itself or even better, before.

I'm certain there will be lots more opportunities to do family things and share intimate escapes, but I need to ensure that my health, wellbeing and sense of self stay strong.

I will give to myself. I will respond to my inner call because I have first-hand experience of what can happen if I don't.

A future message to my beloved family: I love you all, but this is something I need and want to do solo. Sayonara, see you later.

X

Does allocating you-time come easily?

....
....
....

If not, what are some of the excuses you come up with? Once you have written them down examine how unsurmountable these really are.

....
....
....

What is your real reason for not committing to you?

....
....
....

28 July 2011
Journeying to Work

Five weeks and six days after the operation, I drove into work for a few hours. How impressive. My body is amazing! I am in awe of what a wonderful healer my body is: a series of minor miracles reoccurring day in day out. Not only in the physical, but also psychological, emotional and even metaphysical spheres.

I was so grateful to be heading to work, even if only for a few hours. I was ready for a change of scenery and some mental stimulation. Digging out my work bag felt a little weird, and placing some stoma bags into it just in case, even more. I desperately hoped I wouldn't need to do an emergency change in the shared toilet cubicles. I was hit by a surge of nerves just thinking about it.

On my way to university I had the same feeling I get when driving home from the airport after an overseas trip: a little bit of a buzz thinking I am probably the only person on the road returning from whatever distant country I have been in, as most drivers and passengers are in all probability doing a routine trip. So too, on my way to work I gazed at fellow drivers certain I was the only person coming from where I had just been, and I don't mean my home in suburban Carnegie!

I am so blessed to have such a supportive work environment; as my manager says, 'If we can't be supportive in the School of Public Health then there's no hope for anyone!' Colleagues have readily taken on my teaching and marking load and keep reiterating they are happy doing so until I am in better health. Of course this is the way one hopes things should be, but it's certainly not a given, and I for one am not taking it for granted.

So thank you for delivering me safe and sound on this journey, and enabling me to make many, many more journeys, physically and literally.

It is truly wonderful to be alive.

xoxo

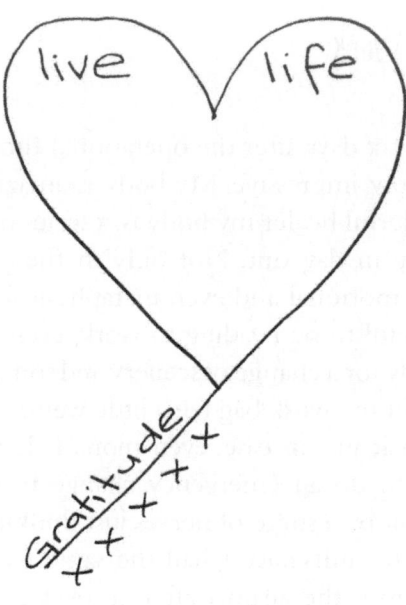

Journal Two

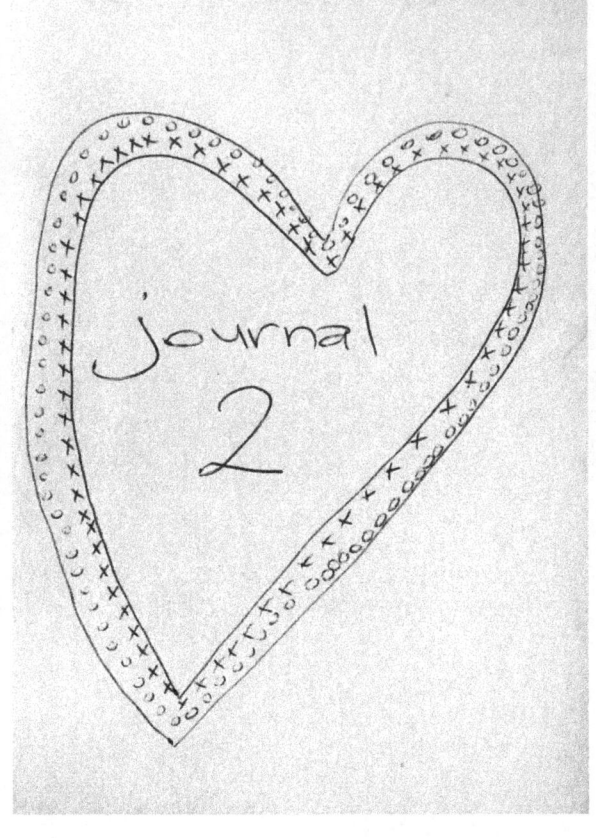

journal
2

10 August 2011

I'm Slipping... No! Don't let apathy creep in!

Isn't it wonderful feeling better? Well of course it is. You can do so much more. Life reverts to a quicker pace and is filled with regular daily routines. Yes, it is absolutely wonderful but ...

What about the daily meditation? OK, what about every second day? No. Well how about weekly? What about those art classes to fill your creative void? What about the writing, the journaling? Ros, what about all those things you promised would become engrained in your new life.

You have to make time! It won't come to you; there will always be other things that need to be done. Remember we've been through this before. Do not let this big lesson be in vain. Do not let those promises you made to yourself become empty ones.

Write

Meditate

Create

Just Do it. No more procrastination or excuses, or there will just be more regret.

I am counting on you to do the right thing—the write thing! A lot of people are counting on me, and I cannot and will not let them down. I owe it to myself. I owe it to them.

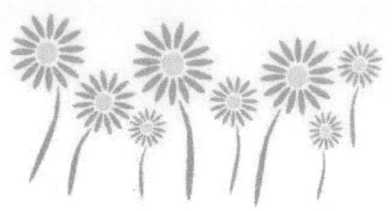

What things do you put off?

....

....

....

What sort of excuses do you come up with?

....

....

....

Do you find it easier coming up with excuses why you can't as opposed to reasons why you can?

....

....

....

What will you do to change?

....

....

....

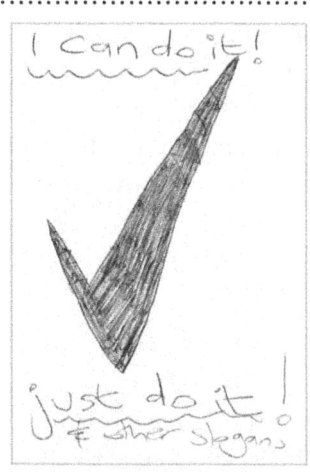

11 August 2011
But she is so young and healthy...

It's remarkable how many times I have heard these words, even thinking them myself. You can't get much healthier than me. I am the brunt of household jokes shunning one piece of chocolate, looking disdainfully at fast food outlets and avoiding snacks between meals. Well sometimes I might snack, but it's always a healthy option: fresh or dried fruit or nuts.

With my slender build, I project an image of good health outwardly, but what does this really tell? It certainly paints a physical landscape, but that's quite different from an emotional one. I may not have fuelled my body with toxic foods (knowingly), but I have struggled with toxic thoughts and emotions. I can excrete foods that disagree with me, but ridding myself of toxic thoughts has always proved more challenging. As my wonderful mother in-law, Lillian, would say, 'All these things Ros, they don't just go to your boots you know'.

Walking slowly around the park, I found myself envying the beautiful gum trees seasonally shedding their skin; I couldn't help but think of the human body and how our cells are renewed every three months. I wondered how we could be truly free of unwanted thoughts, negative emotions, old baggage and the malingering effects of toxic relationships. They float around and haunt us, like an apple bobbing in water, submerging only for a short while before once again popping up to the surface.

Then I remembered the findings of Sonia Lyubomirsky, a behavioural psychologist[4] who says genetics only account for 50% of our wellbeing. Our intentional activity, be it behavioural,

---

4   Lyubomirsky, S., Sheldon, K. M., & Schkade, D. (2005). Pursuing happiness: The architecture of sustainable change. Review of General Psychology, 9, 111-131.

cognitive or motivational makes up another 40% while the last 10% relates to a person's circumstances. We have more control over our life than we dare believe possible. How we respond to a particular situation can be an even greater determinant of our wellbeing than the situation itself. I find this really gratifying and much more empowering. It's really up to us. Do we accept or resist? Do we shrivel or do we grow?

Returning to those external observations, yes, I am young, I do eat healthily, but that does not make me immune to toxicity or negative health events. I would like to believe it minimises them and makes them less severe. Health is such a complex web of social, physical, emotional and even spiritual factors. Even if we think we comprehend contributing factors behind a particular occurrence, we never really know; the best we can do is look for a pattern and hazard a guess. Which doesn't mean I haven't jested about taking up smoking and drinking, eating junk food and partying frequently post diagnosis!

How do people view you?

....
....
....

How do you view yourself?

....
....
....

Is there a big gap between how the outside world views you and the real
you?

....
....
....

If so, whose perspective do you accept more?

....
....
....

20 August 2011

Mummy, why did you get cancer?

12-year-old Zak posed the question, 'Mummy, why did you get cancer?' nine weeks and two days after my operation. Where to begin? It's difficult enough making sense of traumatic life events as an adult, but to a child it can be even harder.

An already anxious and at times fearful child, Danny and I have been noticing some subtle and some more obvious changes in Zak's behaviour that have begun to raise alarm bells.

First it was the incessant, persistent enquiries regarding germs. He would close toilet doors with an outstretched sleeve, study labels on food products checking for expiry dates, scrutinise food for any perceived blemish or imperfection, and spit indiscriminately for no apparent reason. There was also the inability to just settle and drift off to sleep when a string of 'urgent' requests would often appear. Finally he seemed to have developed a slight obsession with his own health, stressing over any and every symptom ranging from a blister to a cough. He would often ask when they would go away and if they ever would!

So, what to make of all of this? A kinesiology appointment three weeks prior left me quietly aghast. The practitioner identified a fear of getting sick and a sub or unconscious belief that cancer was caused through germs. When Zak was questioned about this conviction, out of embarrassment, or perhaps because it really did not resonate, he emphatically stated that, no he didn't believe that was the case.

Next in line was a consultation with the school psychologist who assessed him and mentioned a known condition whereby someone believes they can get transference of cancer through germs. He had yet to treat someone in which this had manifested. Our challenge was his excitement and regular sessions were set up.

But back to the question. During and following gardening today, Zak kept spitting. When asked why, he responded he had dirt in his mouth. Observing him for a while, I noted that in this arduous (not) gardening session barely any dirt had touched his hands, let alone gone anywhere near his mouth. The spitting continued after any remaining dust would have well and truly disappeared.

Preparing dinner, I enlisted his help to ensure the contents of the frying pan did not catch, and asked him why he kept spitting. He replied, 'Germs'. By this stage my calm demeanour was slipping away. Having had several conversations on the topic of germs post-op, I did not anticipate I could shed any new light on this issue. Nonetheless, something prompted me to prod deeper. I told him our bodies were well equipped to deal with germs. Certainly in the instance of dirt, a little bit doesn't hurt, even if it does go into your mouth, you can just rinse your mouth out with water, or have a drink. I then told him about children brought up in homes without pets, in a super-sanitised environment, whose immunity is not as strong as children exposed to some amount of dust, dirt and germs. 'It's what makes our immune system stronger,' I added.

I continued reeling out all things public health until he interrupted, and the conversation abruptly ended with the following, 'I don't want to get cancer.'

Utterly shocked, I responded that you couldn't catch cancer from germs in the most composed manner possible. It can't be spread from one person to another. You can get it as a result of a complex mix of things, such as exposure to certain chemicals, your genes, nutrition (or lack thereof), but you can't catch cancer.

Then his words, 'So why did you get cancer?'

Well, this was one question I had not been anticipating and decided it was high time to turn off the frying pan. I paused momentarily and silently prayed I could do justice to this simply worded, innocent question. I wondered if I would be able to quell his fears and say the right thing. In short I was not sure but responded with great trepidation.

I told him I would probably never know the specific cause, as in all likelihood it was a combination of many things. I was reticent to discuss a likely genetic predisposition to bowel cancer, fearing he would leap to the conclusion that he, being my son, may share this predisposition. So even though in my mind stress was just part of a bigger picture I began recounting things I hoped he couldn't relate back to himself. Moving back from the UK, starting not one but two new jobs in that new year, Dad being away four stints in that year, Granny having a heart attack, a family member's ill health, just to name a few. On reflection perhaps I shouldn't have spouted out all these things, as in some manner these may have impacted on him, but I was so determined to steer his mind away from the germ focus and to be as open and honest as possible.

His response to my deluge, 'Well I have stress in my life too.'

This was not going to be an easily resolved conversation. The more I said, the more I sank. Trying to impart my 40 + year old wisdoms, life philosophies, worldview and rationale for the cancer may have spoken volumes to me, but to Zak I could have been speaking another language. He could only absorb ideas from his point of reference, that of a boy with a total of 12 years of experience. God help me here!

Before addressing his stresses and stressors, I began discussing the social, emotional, physical and nutritional contributors to cancer. cancer had become known as a 'lifestyle' disease with an array of complex causes far beyond stress. It could really symbolise dis-ease at multiple levels. But despite my efforts, my words sounded like 'blah, blah, blah' falling deaf even to my ears. It's one thing to lecture to a bunch of Health Science students; but it's quite another to answer your own son with his innocent gaze shooting searing daggers through your heart and soul.

I asked him to outline his stresses, to which he responded: insufficient chill-out time in front to the TV, being persistently reminded to practice piano and his Bar Mitzvah portion, and walking the dog. He even went to the trouble of recounting the last time he had done so, when a very excited Rufus had discovered a trail of half-eaten bagels on the other side of the park rendering him deaf to Zak's calls of distress.

My words had run dry. All that could be done was to scoop him up into the core of my body and squeeze all the love I had in this world into his.

Now as I write I am considering the big thing he could not vocalise: having to confront the realisation that mum is a mortal being, that we are all mortal beings. Thinking about all the fear residing within his slight, young frame fills me with such sorrow.

My wish for Zak is that he will always be loved deeply and enjoy peace in his inner world, enough to weather the pockets of turbulence that may rise from time to time.

Wishing him much PEACE and LOVE

xxx

Peace of Mind

Peace of Body

Peace of Spirit

Peaceful Soul

Have you ever been stumped, unsure about how to address a particularly sensitive or difficult question? If so, how did you respond? Did it achieve the desired results or make matters worse? A word of warning, before addressing any difficult question, ground yourself. The quickest and most effective way of doing this is by pausing before responding. Take some deep breaths, or even delay your response until you feel ready. Just take your time.

26 August 2011
Loving something for what it is

In hospital, I had calculated how many times I would need to change my stoma bag on the basis of once every two days over a twelve-week period or, for ease of calculation, once a day over six weeks (clever I know!). The result was 42 stomal bag changes minus the four already done in hospital, so 38 times. I purposefully decided against factoring in bag spoilages or other related disasters, abiding to the bare minimum.

I recognised how much psychological strength was required to undergo the operation, and with a similar degree of mental preparation psyched myself up to change bag number 1. It was like I was about to run a marathon. Sleeves rolled up, deep breaths in, internal pep talk, followed by external pep talk. I booted Danny out of the way so I could be totally focused but positioned within shouting range just in case. I was fully aware that if he stayed at my side he would likely pass out, as had previously happened at the cutting of our firstborn's umbilical cord. 'I can do it, I can do it Holsman,' I told myself, incanting my maiden name for added motivation.

Initially I anticipated holding my breath for as long as I could and then optimistically hoped I could get away with just a few more. I prayed that I was indeed up for it. I shouted out for Danny to move closer and then lay out all I needed: the bag, the chux wipes, extra toilet paper. Was there anything else I needed? Ah yes, the disposable nappy bag and adhesive non-alcoholised wipes. I quickly recapped the instructive practice I underwent in hospital. Another quick prayer that this was indeed all I needed.

I questioned how deeply I could really expect my breaths to be when I barely managed superficial ones. There was no point procrastinating anymore. I began self-narrating the instructions, as if I was the stomal nurse, 'OK, you will be fine. Have you got everything you need?'

'OK, let's begin,' I continued. 'Remember, peel the skin away from the adhesive seal, not the adhesive seal away from the skin. Excellent, nearly there. Right, what do you do next? Excellent, the toilet paper. Give it a wipe then dispose in the nappy bag. Did you remember to moisten, not thoroughly wet one of the wipes? Good. Wipe around the exposed area, confidently. Excellent. Remember to lift the stoma so you can wipe around it. Don't be scared! You're doing great. OK, now get the other dry wipe and thoroughly dry the area. Remember, this is really important: if it's still wet, the seal won't be able to adhere.'

The last thing I would have needed or wanted was to go through this traumatic bag change, to just to have to do it all over again. Oh God, please give me strength!

'Right. Back on task. Get the bag. Have you taken off the protective seal? Have you rolled the end of the bag and sealed it closed? Yes, great. You are doing really well!'

'Almost there,' I went on, 'OK so lift the top area of skin above the stoma to make it easier to fit the bag. Great. Now make sure the bottom of the bag is at a good angle: pointing more or less midway between your legs to ensure an easier emptying process. Fantastic. Ros you are doing so well! Now rub the adhesive area well with the non-alcohol adhesive wipes and make sure there are no air bubbles or you could get a leak. A leak will find and follow the path of least resistance. The warmth of your skin will help.'

So pressing and gently caressing the seal, I once again hoped and prayed that all would be fine. I coped with the smell, I coped with the physical look of my protruding bowel,.

I had done it! I shouted down the corridor to Danny that all was well. I felt the need to wipe my brow given the amount of stress I had just undergone and level of endurance required to complete it. All that was missing were beads of sweat; they were on the inside, contained behind my brow. This was definitely the closest I had ever got to completing a marathon!

Once again I calculated how many more to go? Good Lord, how will I be able to endure so many more? How stressful. How time consuming. The sight of the full nappy bag, once again reminding me I was like a baby reborn again, feeling vulnerable and dependent, but in another way quite accepting of my new temporary reality.

Aware of the impact of my thoughts on how things play out, I tried speaking kindly about my stoma during the next few weeks. At my first appointment with the oncology psychologist, I piped up saying, 'I can't say I love my stoma.' It was amazing, as soon as these words left my mouth, feelings of guilt suddenly flooded my consciousness. I had visions of punitive measures in the form of blockages that I had been forewarned about. I then acknowledged it was OK for me not to love my stoma; it was only temporary and was playing an important role, optimising healing in the operated area.

Ten or so weeks down the track to the present moment, I am filled by amazement at what my body has gotten used to. I still can't say I'm in love with my stoma, but I can say I love certain aspects of it. I have not had to concern myself about the effects of certain foods playing havoc on my system, as it is physically impossible to get constipated with an ileostomy. I have even enjoyed a wider range of foods, such as cheese which I avoided pre-op. I am on a restrictive low-fibre diet, so I can't have a diverse spread of fruit, vegetables and legumes that would ordinarily have formed a large percentage of my diet, but the novelty of eating more fattening, sugary, low-fibre foods, that for so many years I have shunned, is strangely appealing. Breads, potatoes, pasta, cakes, muffins fuel my slender body and amuse my pre-programmed, health-food-cued brain.

The more I think about it, the more I love it. It's actually quite liberating, and while it might make me feel a little nauseated one day, or make my 'outputs' (as they have been referred to) more runny, it's not nearly as bad as the cramping, diarrhoea and constipation I endured for so long. I have come to realise that having a shorter passage of time between eating food and it passing from my system is a blessing in disguise.

I am even becoming much braver, daring to shower without

the bag, delicately washing the stoma with my fingers under running water; even the sight of it protruding from my skin does not sicken me as it once did. I now wonder what it will be like to regain full function of my rectum and anus. Sure I have had the urge and even on occasion have dreamt of doing a poo—yes that's right, through my anus and directly into the toilet bowl. How extraordinary life is; losing the function of my anus for three whole months, something I would never in a million years contemplated some five months ago, and why would I?

Now I nervously anticipate the return of normal bowel function, scheduled in just under two weeks! What a journey. I certainly won't be writing any farewell messages on the bag for the surgeon to muse on, like a woman I met who underwent the same operation. She recounted that in the short time she had the bag, she could not bond with it. Donning a surgical mask for bag changes, she hurried the reversal period, refusing to have it any longer than the bare minimum of eight weeks. I have to admit I am quite proud of how I have bonded with it. Admittedly it was far from an easy beginning, but what new challenge ever is?

I have so much to be grateful for. It has enabled me to have a quality of life in the last two months I don't think I would have been able to have. Of course I will be delighted to regain the flat surface of my stomach, have a long soak in a hot bath and regain my wardrobe, which, for these past couple of months, has mimicked a pregnancy wardrobe—a few new items of clothing with appropriately giving waistlines worn in a combination of mix and match options. I also won't miss the embarrassing cacophony of sounds emitted from the bag, like gumboots squelching in mud.

How strange to be thinking of a return to normalcy. I am certainly devoting more time thinking about this than I ever did about having an artificial bottom.

Thank you stoma for helping my bowel heal. May my first experience utilising normal bowel function be a good one and may I continue to heal, improve and strengthen.

xoxo

Has there been something in your life that you have come around to loving or appreciating when your initial feeling was of rejection, conflict, distance or animosity?

....

....

....

What helped you change? Time? What else?

....

....

....

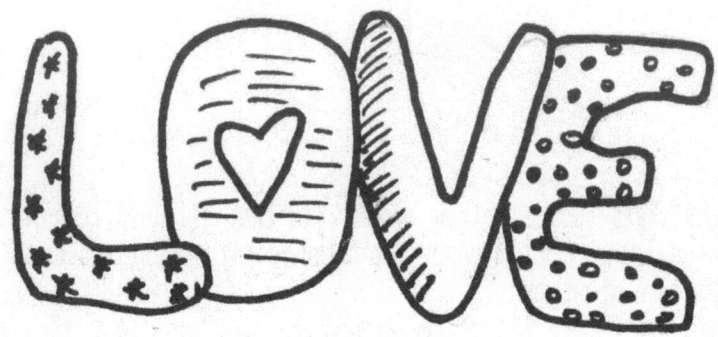

Not I love you, or he loves me — just "LOVE" in its own right.

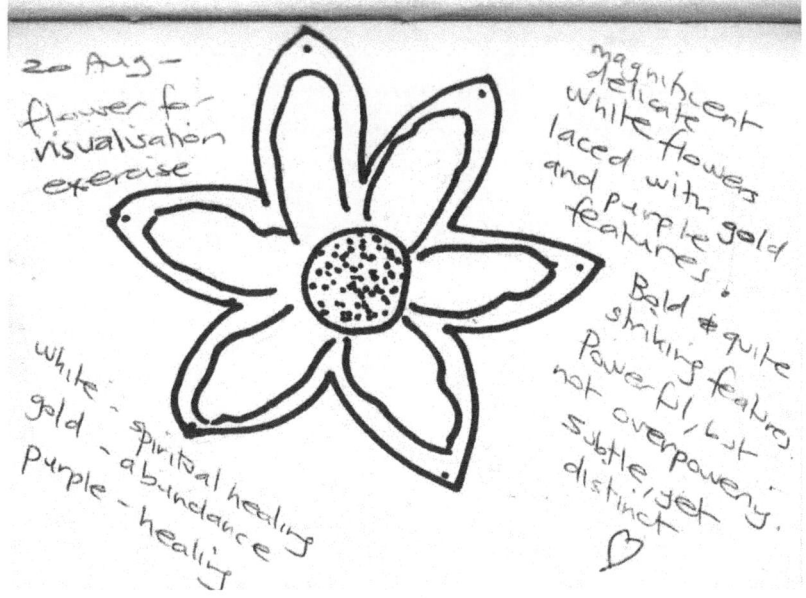

20 Aug — flower for visualisation exercise

magnificent delicate white flowers laced with gold and purple features.

Bold & quite striking features. Powerful, but not overpowering. Subtle, yet distinct ♡

white — spiritual healing
gold — abundance
purple — healing

3 September 2011
Changing your life at traffic lights

When I was an undergraduate student, the people closest to me used to joke that I must be completing assignments at traffic lights. Running from here to there and everywhere other than university, it seemed the only plausible explanation for my better-than-expected grades. Note to my students, past and present: please do not read the above paragraph, and if you have, do not take it as sound advice. Move on and ignore!

I put in the bare minimum of effort, only occasionally attending tutorials or lectures (I am cringing writing this!). Life outside university was vastly more exciting. A hectic social life infused with a great sense of purpose and responsibility as a youth movement leader. I willingly spent countless hours dreaming up inspirational weekly programs, planning for summer and winter camps and scheduling agendas for national and federal meetings.

Those preparations were rarely conducted at traffic lights. Had I spent one-tenth of the time I freely devoted to my youth movement and social life on my university work, I probably would have excelled. Alas, it was not meant to be. So seemingly slack that as the end first year approached my dad made a bet with me: if I passed he would pay my fare to England to visit my then boyfriend, Danny. This was a bet I couldn't refuse, bearing no consequence or payback other than a potential dint to my ego. My dad rested, reassured it would be one of the safest bets he would ever make.

Six weeks later I excitedly crossed half the globe, courtesy of Dad. He never, ever, made a bet with me (or anyone else) again!

Whether in my DNA or through life's programming, I have always been a speedy Gonzales, racing around, doing things quickly. My mother-in-law marvels as I whip up a storm:

chopping, frying, and assembling an array of dishes for diverse dietary palates, including vegan, vegetarian and outright fussy. I dart from place to place, ticking chores off my list while dropping off and collecting children from school, and taking on extra-curricular activities and play dates.

I am a quick thinker, quick doer and quick-acting person, which comes with distinct bonuses but also several drawbacks. I have learnt at my expense that slow thinking, slow doing and slow acting also goes a long way.

Anyway, as a pre-programmed quick person, I love quick fixes: a little bit here, a little bit there, minus a portion of dedicated commitment and diligence. I misguidedly believed everything could be done at a pace: child rearing, career, hobbies, you name it. I would zip through all the procedural steps, blinkered to signs of fatigue and stress, somehow convincing myself these to be quite 'normal' and 'not so bad'. After all, I rationalised, with a history of chronic fatigue syndrome, I couldn't expect my energy levels to be great, not to mention the fact I was not getting any younger.

Over the years, as my grey hairs started taking root, I began questioning my flawed logic. I recognised the need to slow down. But when you're born running it's easier said than done. If only I had learnt this in my earlier years, at school for example, but on reflection maybe it's something we need to learn on our own, slowly and surely in small deliberate steps, not leaps and bounds.

So how does one transition from hare to tortoise? Countless hours spent on the couch quarantined my body and grew my mind. If doing things at traffic lights was my innate strength, perhaps I could use it to my advantage and apply the 'Traffic Light Principle' to my life. Life is busy. Life is hectic. Days are filled with many things that all compete for our time.

Now after years and years of oblivion, it has suddenly dawned on me. I need to bring a level of conscious awareness into my day to signal when to slow down and when to stop, to bring my racing body to an enforced halt through scheduled quietness and stillness.

This can be activated at any time of day and doesn't even require a perfect Zen setting, as sometimes that's just not possible.

Within us resides a special sanctuary: our inner Temple of peace, harmony and inner reflection. It's just a matter of tapping into it. Even traffic lights can be the best place to rekindle this awakening. The best place, because you're sitting idling with time on your hands, and that's all you need.

So when you're next at a traffic light, feeling hot under the collar, become mindful of your inner sanctuary.

Smile

Breathe

Say your affirmations

Short of burning an incense stick to conjure up a meditative, peaceful atmosphere, you will be amazed at how great a shift in energy is, without even moving from the seat of your car. Just please don't close your eyes during this process!

Visualise the red traffic light sending you powerful regenerative and restorative energy. Followed by the amber light signalling transition to green, when you are ready to go.

You have been revived. You have received energy. For that one moment, rather than feeling frustrated by being slowed down with the interruption of a red light, surrender to this pause. Give something back to yourself. Bolster the universal life force that exists within you. It's always present. Just become aware of it. Let the traffic light tap into this consciousness. Breathe it in. Breathe it out.

Whilst this sanctuary resides externally we can always come up with excuses: too noisy, not the right place, too many other things competing for my time and so on. Yet if the sanctuary is within, there can be no excuses. Like an internal pop up tent, all you need is a mental stimulus such as an affirmation, smile, thought pattern, or even some deep breaths and your sanctuary will instantly be erected whether you are stuck in traffic, in a long boring meeting, or even in your living room with household noises.

Use those traffic light moments to connect to your inner sanctuary, slow down, regenerate and regain focus. Now you are ready to travel safe and protected on your journey, both in the car and beyond.

X

Breathe in deeply and focus your attention on the different colours of the traffic light:

- **Red:** Root chakra (base of your spine)
- **Orange:** Sacral chakra (pelvic area)
- **Green:** Heart chakra

Breathe in the red for a count of 5, hold for a count of 5 then exhale for a count of 5.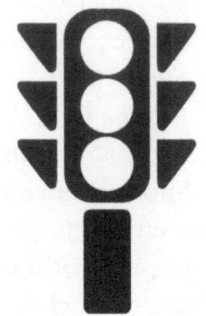
Repeat this rhythmic breathing for the duration of the traffic light until it's green and you're ready to go.
You will be disappointed the light doesn't stay red longer!

A Note about Chakras

Within the body there are a series of minor and major energy centres called chakras. Chakra is the Sanskrit word for "wheel" or "disk". Each of these chakras has its own distinct character and relates to a unique aspect of our being. Chakras correlate to levels of consciousness, body functions, colours, elements and even sounds. The seven major chakras are located alongside the spine following a central energy line. It is believed that blocked energy in our chakras can lead to illness. The seven chakras are:

Crown		**Heart**	
Colour:	Purple	Colour:	Green
Element:	Spirituality	Element:	Love / Healing
Third Eye		**Solar Plexus**	
Colour:	Indigo	Colour:	Yellow
Element:	Awareness	Element:	Wisdom / Power
Throat		**Sacral**	
Colour:	Blue	Colour:	Orange
Element:	Communication	Element:	Sexuality / Creativity
		Root	
		Colour:	Red
		Element:	Basic trust

10 September 2011

Words harm, words heal

I'm thinking a lot about my impending bowel reversal, pondering on the word reversal. For added clarity I seek out a dictionary: A change in an opposite direction or course of action; an unfortunate happening that hinders or impedes; something that is thwarting or frustrating. Out of curiosity, I right-click to bring up a lengthy list of synonyms: setback, hitch, blow, snag, misfortune, difficulty, turn around, U-turn.

I'm struck by the negative slant in these definitions. Before all this happened, I doubt I would have ever given the word reversal, let alone its negative connotations, much consideration. But here I am, pondering over the term's inherent implications of going backwards.

I don't want things to go back to the way they were; after all, it is this former state of things that might have contributed to the cancer diagnosis in the first place. I want to return to newness, to a new beginning. The old is well and truly gone. I've been blessed with a whole new rectum: an entirely new replacement part that has left me feeling slightly bemused and, if I'm honest, a little bit freaked out! Man-made godliness resides within.

My bowel will be stitched up and rerouted. It's not a step backwards, but a faintly familiar path untrodden in over three months. It has been rid of a noxious self-sown weed, now clear of negativity and toxicity.

Word choice really is important. You only need to think of how much time and energy advertising and marketing companies invest on words: words to appeal, to create a need or desire for a product, to make you feel better about yourself. So why not invest some time infusing them with positivity?

Now I'm thinking of all those catch phrases we recite without questioning that contain so much negativity: chocolate to die for, hugged to death, drop-dead gorgeous, I love you to death, deadlines, too much of a good thing, etc. Isn't it strange that we don't hear the opposite? Chocolate to live for, hugged to life, stay-alive gorgeous, I love you to life, lifelines, You can never have too much of a good thing!

What a shame the medical fraternity has chosen such negative terminology to describe this procedure. It really doesn't sit well with me. I am choosing to rephrase this procedure with a positive mindset. I need to do this for myself. Words harm, but they also have the potential to heal.

A bowel reconnection. Intuitively it sounds so much better.

Now back to the dictionary. To reconnect: connect back together; establish a bond of communication or emotion; to provide a service, such as water, electricity or the telephone after they have been disconnected. And as for those synonyms: rewire, rejoin, recouple, relink, recombine. All inherently positive!

Rather than using a term associated with a reversal of fortune, or going backwards, I am hereby declaring I will refer to this procedure from a more positive viewpoint. I am going to have a bowel reconnection. That's what is happening!

Like a dear friend who has parted ways due to life circumstances and then wondrously reconnected, so too will the two ends of my bowel. They may need some time to get reacquainted, to feel comfortable in one another's company, but at the end of the day this is a reconnection to familiar territory. These won't be strangers having to start from an awkward or unknown vantage point.

It's amazing how in mulling this over I feel so much lighter and brighter. The feelings of anguish and nervousness that lay in the pit of my stomach less than 20 minutes ago have been usurped by hope and excitement.

I am so grateful I have taken time to embrace my 'reconnection' and reframe it in my own language.

The language of love
The language of optimism
The language of love (yes love!)

The term reconnection conjures up happy times, shared bonds, a blending of histories and tenderness of emotions. My bowel will be reconnected. It will know what to do like two hands reaching for each other in the dark. Reunited on a common path, bound together for the journey ahead.

xox

Words are loaded with emotion. Some positive, some negative. Think about some of the words you use and how they make you feel.

....

....

....

Do they have a negative or positive charge? How could you rephrase these into more positive ones?

....

....

....

Have you had (or will you be having) an operation or procedure with a name that makes you feel uneasy? Think of another name that sits better with you.

....

....

....

19 September 2011

These are a few of my favourite things

Some things you can't ever imagine not being able to do. I'm wistfully recollecting the many things I have dreamt I could do post-surgery in no particular order:

1. Lying on my stomach
2. Taking a deep, long, relaxing bath
3. Wearing my jeans, not some temporary wide-waisted ring-ins
4. Making love skin-to-skin, not skin-to-bag-to-skin
5. Embracing family and friends without a disquieting feeling they may become aware of my protruding bag
6. And it has to be said, sitting on the toilet and doing a poo!

These are all things I have taken for granted in the past. There have been other times in my life when wearing tightly fitted jeans or lying on my stomach for rests became impossible, but that was due to a pregnant belly swollen with a new life, and not a bulging stoma bag filled with excrement. Oh, to lie on my stomach, face down on the shaggy living room carpet, with the sun streaming in on my back. My ideal power nap.

And baths. There's nothing better than a long soak at the end of a stress-filled day, as muscle tension dissolves into the steamy hot water inducing immediate relaxation; a touch of luxury well within reach, so blissful yet so utterly decadent. But it's just not possible with a stoma bag. I'm so grateful this is temporary, and I've great empathy, and sympathy, for those with more permanent fixtures. I at least have a countdown.

As for making love skin-to-skin, what a test this whole episode has been to intimacy and our marriage as a whole! After the operation, the last thing I had imagined was that the desire to make love would return, but, much like after childbirth, over time it does. Such a bizarre concept: making love separated by a stoma bag. It has to be said, it definitely grosses me out, and I would imagine Danny feels similarly, but as they say in the classics 'Life goes on'. I just never imagined it would go on like this.

When a few weeks ago the twinge of amorousness returned, the surgeon's words rang in my ears. Will it feel any different? Will there be pain or discomfort? I just had to know and broached the subject with Danny. He was willing to give it a go. Danny deserves a medal for the patience he has displayed not just recently but on and off over many years. Ever so tentatively we made love. Even though there may not have been fireworks, re-establishing intimacy was so important. To be enveloped in my beloved's embrace, even with the intrusion of a towel pressed against his skin in an attempt to disguise the disquieting bulge, felt so good. I tentatively asked Danny if it felt any different, but he didn't think so. Such a relief. The thought of losing or having altered sexual function would have been a huge sacrifice to bear, and blessedly not one I had to make. All is well. I am so incredibly blessed to have a life partner who, strange as it may seem, loves and finds me attractive, even when an alarming bag protrudes from my belly. If that's not love then what is?

As for other less intimate embraces, I am quite self-conscious, not just of the bulge, but also of the disquieting noises the bag produces. I feel more comfortable in noisier places, hugging chest to chest, as opposed to a full bear hug. I love bear hugs! But any form of embrace is good for the soul and I am so grateful to the many hugs that have been endowed on me these past few months in particular.

The real adjustment has been retraining my mind to accept that as long as I am fitted with this bag, no matter how long I sit on the toilet, nothing will happen, no number two! It has been a real void in my daily ritual, a part of my routine since being toilet-trained as a toddler. Come rain, shine or fall, no matter our cultural background or skin colour it's what we all do: eliminate waste naturally.

I wonder what it will be like to once again indulge in these things. How long will it be before I take them for granted as I have done over a lifetime? Or will I promise to appreciate these things, to treasure, graciously savour and warmly welcome them back into my habituated life? Who knows. If I'm feeling really decadent perhaps I will even indulge in multiple activities in the one day: wear my snugly fitted jeans, share a bear hug with a friend, sneak a nap on my stomach in the middle of the day, squeeze in a toilet stop when the urge arises, as nature intended, and end my day with a long soak in a hot bath followed by making love.

Bliss! X

List three of your favourite things.

....
....
....

Has there been a time you had to do without these?

....
....
....

When once again these things became accessible, did you all-too-soon take them for granted?

....
....
....

19 September 2011

From lashing out to loving in

It amazes me that even after this experience, I still persist in thinking that putting up an internal fight somehow helps. I naturally gravitate towards resisting something rather than accepting it.

My countdown is in full swing. Only two days until my bowel reconnection. Danny returned from his two-week filming jaunt in Lithuania and I greeted him unenthusiastically with an unmistakably sore throat. The last thing I want is to get sick.

I am annoyed at each and every person crossing my path. At Zak for sharing this bug. At Danny for being absent and now jetlagged, rendering him incompetent of anything aside from falling asleep on the couch. At Josh. Well, just about everyone and everything.

Woe is me. I'm having another operation and people are just not giving me the sympathy and attention I deserve. Out with friends for lunch, the conversation revolves around shoes, camping equipment, and so on. Hello, what about what I have been going through? Anyone interested in that?

Fatigue mounts, as does the lump in my throat. I wince with each and every swallow. This is just not supposed to be. My op is in two days. I'm entrenched by inflexible, intransigent and negative thoughts. When the potential to see the positive side of postponing the operation arises I instantly resist. No, I don't want to think of any positive reasons. I want to sulk. I want to wallow and make everyone around me, myself included, suffer.

Finally I take leave of my negative stream of consciousness and find a nice sunny spot indoors to snooze. Everyone has been forewarned. No distractions. No disruptions and NO noise.

Soon, anger and frustration give way to gentle waves of relaxation. Then seemingly metres away a child screams while running past our house and I am jolted into full consciousness, once again irritated. I try to return to my peaceful dwelling space. I toss, I turn, I inhale deeply, but to no avail. My peace is gone.

The virus has seeped deeper inside my head, bones and muscles. I resolve to be a better person to those I love. I try to be nice. I try to be interested in what they were doing, but it is an uphill battle.

I was on strike. No, I wouldn't make dinner. No, no, and no! Takeaway was ordered. After dinner we opted for family TV time and chose the IT Crowd, a comedy. The four of us squeezed onto our 3-seater couch and in no time at all I was lost in laughter. I felt a shift inside. It felt great. We were all sniggering, guffawing and laughing together as one and it was the best feeling ever! Even though it still hurt to swallow I was loving every second of this shift into light-heartedness.

Bedtime fast approached and I kissed everyone goodnight with genuine affection (whilst trying not to breathe my germs onto them). I couldn't apologise for the darkened mood that consumed me before, but I could end the day on a brighter note. With a smile on my face I turned out the light knowing that whatever the outcome of my virus, tomorrow would be a better, brighter day.

Skip ahead nine glorious hours…I lifted my head from the pillow noting that although physically it was loaded with mucous, I was strangely at peace and inwardly lighter. Thankfully I had woken up on the right side of the bed. Early indicators certainly seemed optimistic.

I knew what I had to do: call the surgeon and postpone the op for a few days. Intuitively and instinctively I knew this to be the right decision. Unlike yesterday where the mere thought of postponement brought up a tidal wave of resistance and resentment, I actually felt great. One phone call later I was informed that postponing was not an issue, but due to the late notice I had three options:

1. Go ahead with the operation tomorrow even though I was not feeling 100% (to say the least)

2. Have the operation the following week, one day before Rosh Hashanah.

3. Have the operation Monday fortnight.

I asked to speak to the surgeon directly as there was one thing I had been hesitating about. I explained to him about our still to be confirmed trip to Israel for Zak's Bar Mitzvah as I thought some additional recovery time may be beneficial. He responded that two or three weeks later would not make much difference to a planned trip in January.

So focused on making a decision for three months hence, and in my impatience to rid myself of this bag, I had almost forgotten the importance of taking care of myself in the here and now. Adding to this I was overlooking two very important occasions: my mum's 80th birthday this very Sunday and Rosh Hashanah (Jewish New Year) the following week. A while ago, as a family, we decided to postpone the 80th celebrations for a couple of weeks. 'It was just one of those things,' I rationalised, knowing in my heart of hearts it would not have been the same.

Decision made. It was a no brainer. I was going to celebrate mum's 80th and Rosh Hashanah with friends and family, then have the operation in the lead up to the days of introspection prior to Yom Kippur (the Day of Atonement). How apt.

By this stage my voice had grown huskier and head heavier but I was enlivened by my decision. To celebrate! There is a time for everything and the next two weeks would be filled with joy and a celebration of life.

Reinvigorated and buoyed by optimism, I felt the need to commune with nature and suggested to Danny we head to the Yarra River for lunch and a walk, something that had been farthermost from my mind less than 24 hours ago. Sitting underneath an aged gum munching away on lunch, I marvelled at its growth and form. Wrinkled smooth bark wrapped not only around the older branches but also the younger, more slender ones. They were absolutely beautiful. I began reflecting on how, in our youth and beauty-obsessed culture, people go to great lengths to eradicate wrinkles and sagging skin from external view. What a shame, I thought. In these wrinkles is a lifetime of experiences. What's so bad about that? They are a physical reminder of our true selves and what a privilege it is to grow old enough to have them.

Now I was feeling so grateful to have caught this virus. It helped me focus on the present and enjoy the moment. I also learnt that my sister Natalie intended to surprise mum and would be flying in from New York in a few days. It would be one of only a few occasions where the entire family would be together and what a present that was for mum. All four children under the same roof at the same time, honouring our mum: the family matriarch.

At home, I thanked Zak for sharing his virus with me and told him how grateful I was that as a result I would be able to celebrate Granny's 80th and Rosh Hashanah. His philosophical, mature response took me by surprise, especially considering he had recently seemed more like 12 going on 5 than 12 going on 55!

'So now you can be happy and replenished and then have your operation,' he remarked.

And he was absolutely right!

So thank you universe for putting in my path a blessing disguised as an obstacle. It enabled me to make the decision not only best for me but best for everyone.

Do you tend to accept or resist newly presented challenges?

....

....

....

If you are a resister, what strategies can you think of to help you shift to a place of acceptance?

....

....

....

People heal better when there's less internal resistance and it certainly makes for a calmer life — and I'm talking from experience!

26 September 2011

Extra time

This virus really was heaven-sent. What was I thinking, denying myself the celebration of these precious moments for the sake of a few less days with the stoma bag and few more days recovering prior to our still unconfirmed trip in January?

It feels like I've been granted extra time. Today I was meant to be in hospital but instead was at Josh's end of semester musical soiree. Propped up with pillows in a hospital bed I missed his last performance three months ago. Now I am seven rows from the front of the stage, beaming from ear to ear, not only in response to the talented musical performances but also in my own body. It too has excelled in healing and delivered a masterful performance. I am so incredibly grateful to be part of this audience and experience.

Mum turned 80 on Sunday 25 September. What a milestone. She has come such a long way since she and her family fled the glass and blood-strewn streets of Nazi Germany. Her personal and professional achievements have been great, although, humble and modest as she is, I know she would beg to differ. Now as she steadily slips into the fearsome terrain of Alzheimer's, she is most content at my dad's side. What a cruel and undignified disease, to put it mildly. From an external eye, all things considered, she seems to be doing OK, still living independently under the increasing intervention and watchful eye of my father's doting hands. Yet, I'm already mourning the person she once was. Physically she is present, but her once highly capable persona is largely absent— an inferior replica, but still my mum.

Her birthday was for her an almost surreal experience, partly because her mind was taking a slow leave of absence but also in the recognition that she was reaching an age that seems reserved for other people. Asking how she felt, she replied, 'Overcome,' which I thought a very apt word choice, especially as expressing herself has become such a challenge. Other words began forming but evaporated before her lips could release them. Frustration rather than consonants and vowels filled the air. I think I too would be overcome. In any case what single word best describes waking up as a first-time octogenarian?

What a glorious day: the extended family, idyllic blue sky, spring air warmed by gentle rays of sunshine, not yet tinted by the harshness of summer and Natalie's presence. I only recently learnt she booked a frequent flyer ticket long before any of us knew what lay in store.

Buzzing inside with excitement at being able to celebrate this wonderful occasion, not even my croaky voice or tissues bulging inside my sleeve dampened my mood. I was getting such a kick from the knowledge that all four of us 'kids' were together. Unlike some families whose lives overlap and intermingle, this really was a rare and precious occasion. In fact I'm struggling to recall the last time this would have happened. Surely it could not have been almost 20 years ago at our wedding? Surely not? But it was!

The baby of the family with a large age gap between myself and my siblings, I had felt like an only child for a large chunk of my childhood. Peter went interstate to study medicine when he was 19 (I was 6), Natalie for the most part lived away from home after becoming an ultra-orthodox Jew when she was 18 (I was 9), and Emily left home at 21 when I was only 10. Four very different souls, born of one womb, celebrating not only the birthday of our mother but our shared bond together, forever as siblings.

With so few nuclear family memories, this was a truly standout day, exceptionally special and really couldn't have been better. Thank you, thank you, and thank you.

Happy 80th birthday to my beloved mum!

Words cannot express how much love and gratitude
I have for you. Your heart is filled with love and your
actions motivated by kindness.

Wishing you abundant love, laughter
and good health
now and always
xoxoxo

(On 28 May 2014, my beautiful mother passed away aged 82.
I miss her every day. She was a generous and kind-hearted
gentlewoman who loved to smile and laugh, even after her speech
had departed. Her family meant the world to her and she meant
the world to me.)

27 September 2011

Password Changes

Every three months warning messages rudely flash on my Outlook email account. Is it really that time already? I marvel at time's passing. For me, quarterly password changes signal a mini ending of an era and provide an opportunity to set a different tone and intention for my next life-phase.

Although with each and every warning message, the pressure mounts. 'Your password will expire in 10 days. Would you like to change it now?' Each time I ask myself if I'm ready to lock in a new password. Will it be the best choice of word (and numeric value) and intention for the next 12 weeks? Is the trigger associated with this word powerful enough? Is it positive enough? After all, this will be the word I will be reminded of each and every time I log on to my work emails, often countless times in a day, each time impressing a little deeper into my sub-conscious and conscious mind. So, it has to be just right.

I tried remembering former passwords and am surprised at how quickly they vanish from memory. Laughter 1, Happiness 8, Fulfilled 8, Success 120, Robust 18. I felt myself gravitating to Wellbeing 8, but I needed to sit with it first. Crazy as it might sound I actually get a tinge of nervous apprehension before my next password change.

With closure of the ileostomy loop coming up so soon, what should I choose? It could be any previous passwords pertaining to wellbeing or happiness with different numeric values, but I kept revisiting the need for it to be tied to my hopes and desired wishes for the next few months. Words come, words go. Then like a bolt of lightning Reconnect 1 came to mind. I contemplated whether it should be Reconnect 1 or 8, but settled on 1 representing wholeness.

Sitting in front of the computer at work with a heavy head and tissues strewn all over my desk, the warning message once again flashed impatiently on my screen, as did another message reminding me of an imminent meeting. With only one day remaining to change it without any additional complications I hurriedly took the plunge. With a CTRL, ALT, DELETE, I changed my password and entered Connection 1. Something didn't feel quite right. It somehow seemed incomplete, but my colleague was demanding my attention so I was compelled to think about other more pressing matters.

Later that evening at a school concert I saw a familiar face, someone I recognised from a long time ago, but whose name and specific association escaped me. Thankfully in the intermission our eyes met and we shared a warm mutual wave of recognition. We soon realised our parents used to be friendly, and she had attended Sunday school with one of my sisters. It was really lovely seeing her after so many years. Driving home I was filled with warmth thinking about this old friendship, and then it dawned on me I had stuffed up the password. The pressure had got to me. It was meant to be Reconnection 1, not Connection 1. This chance reconnection reminded me of this and so perfectly encapsulated my feelings and intent for the next few months.

What type of passwords do you use? Functional? Intentional? Positive, negative or neutral?

....
....
....

Take some time now to think up a really great affirmations/passwords

....
....
....

7 October 2011

The Countdown has begun

When I was younger I would express my excitement about a particular event or milestone saying 'X' many sleeps to go. Even as an adult sometimes I revert to this measurement of time: 'X' many sleeps until we go away, 'X' many sleeps until Josh or Zak return from camp and so on.

Now with only five more bag changes to go, I am excited, tinged with a smidgeon of nervousness. It is so hard to believe that nearly four months have passed since the momentous first operation, since the fear, doubt and anxiety, and being fitted with a purpose-built new rectum. Now I am an expert bag changer, regularly emptying its contents, whether in the brightness of day or wee hours of the night.

There is such a different feel about this op to the last one. Although pangs of anxiety puncture my inner being (and physical body) from time to time, it is totally different to the anguish and torment I faced four months ago. My most recent bout of nerves prompted me to compose a long list of jet setting/travel destinations that I intend to place prominently on the fridge, like a reverse insurance policy that I'm very much looking forward to expending.

Sure, I'm wondering how my bowel will function, how long it will take to achieve optimal healing, how long I will be in hospital and what my recovery will be like. Will I have much pain? Will I experience nausea? How will the anaesthetic go? Despite the many questions, I am facing this operation from a position of strength and with a degree of confidence. I can see how well my body responded and healed in the past and I know that, whatever the outcome, I will excel in accelerating and optimising my own healing. I am literally being reconnected with a 'closure of the ileostomy loop' as specified on the hospital admission forms. I am getting closure and it's getting close. Really close.

I am ready to put all of this behind me. I commit to directing my affirmations and resolutions towards a fulfilled, healthy and rewarding life ahead.

Whilst in reflection on Yom Kippur (Day of Atonement) I came up with a great acronym, VIP: Vitality, Inspiration, Prosperity. I am a VIP: vital, inspired and prosperous.

My life will be filled with health, vitality and the inspiration to pursue my dreams, ambitions and prosperity in more than just a financial sense. I have to thank God for sealing me in the Book of Life, not the Book of Survival. I promise to live, not merely survive. I promise to contribute, to make a difference and be a source of support to others going through similar or other challenging life experiences. I will go from strength to strength. I am a VIP!

I am going from strength to strength. I don't need ill health to grow. I give myself permission to grow from a perspective of strength, positivity, good and goodness. I owe it to myself. I don't have to be a martyr. I also owe it to Danny and my beautiful boys, Josh and Zak. I look forward to being granted ongoing and multiple blessings and embracing great health, energy and vitality.

I commit to truly living the rest of my days. I summon the assistance from all my guides, spiritual advisors and angels to guide and support me; to be there when I need them and to protect not only myself but also my whole family. With all this love I know I will be fine.

I am ready for closure. I am ready to be reconnected to who I truly am: a giving, loving and healthy woman. And to this I say
Amen.

X X X X

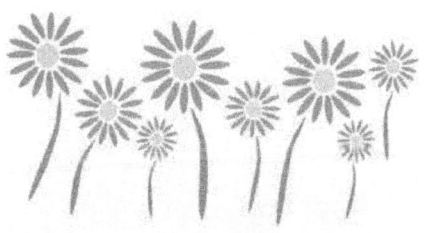

Come up with a much better title than 'Bucket List' and list all the destinations you'd like to visit. Then place it somewhere visible and look forward to ticking as many of these off as you can.

12 October 2011 (Josh's 16th Birthday)
It's Done — CLOSURE

Day 2 post-op and other than nausea I am doing really well. The best thing is I am comfortable enough to breathe and laugh. What a different kind of operation, thank God.

I have returned to the same ward, but have swapped my mountain view for a city outlook. Not sure if there is any symbolism here, but at face value it seems like serenity and calmness has been replaced by action and dynamism, implying a return to an active full life. Bring it on!

There has been great excitement over my passing of wind by nursing staff, with celebrations and even real applause akin to, and perhaps even surpassing, the passing of wind in a new baby.

Talking about new babies, exactly 16 years ago, I was also in hospital giving birth to my gorgeous Josh. What a different hospital adventure that was! Birth, rebirth and life's journey, all deep, mysterious and awesome concepts. That was exciting hospital time. Now I am just grateful not to be in pain and to have returned to familiar surrounds, with the same friendly staff, many of whom were here on my first stay. They really are exceptional here. It has been a bit like a reunion; something I never would have expected. The cleaning staff, food monitors, assorted nurses and ward administrators have welcomed me back with such warmth and delight I have returned for closure.

There must have been countless numbers of people in and out of this ward. It goes to show how making an effort (both ways) to smile, enquire about someone's wellbeing, say hello, display appreciation and demonstrate gratitude; how all these things etch you warmly in someone's mind. Then all that's required is a small spark to reignite these feelings, rekindle the connection and open up the possibility for many more. How wonderful to have been blessed with a sunny disposition, I don't know where I'd be without it. It also seems that the nursing profession has a disproportionately high number of sunny-siders, and for that I am eternally grateful.

Do you find it easy connecting to strangers?

....

....

....

Sharing a smile with someone is one of the most powerful connective tools in human existence. Even if it takes you a little out of your comfort zone, why not share one with someone today?

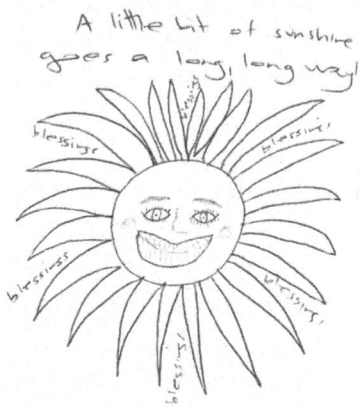

17 October 2011

Be careful what you wish for...

For months I have been dreaming of doing a poo, interspersed with anxieties about whether it would work and if I would feel any different. Post-op, there have been daily questionings and checklists about my anal emissions: wind, old gunky stinky stuff, new stuff, etc.

Day three after the operation, the hospital staff rated me as a 2/3, but in order to go home I needed to open my bowels. Thankfully my appetite was improving and I could feel the increasingly weighty load slowly making its way through my system. Alas, it stopped shy of evacuation.

I wanted to go home tomorrow, 4 nights post-op. The surgeon suggested a laxative if by mid-afternoon there was no action. The urge increased, but still no action.

At 5pm, I asked the nurse for her opinion, mindful of my sensitive system and lighter than average body weight, as to whether a smaller than the recommended dose of laxative might be a better idea. 'No,' she kindly replied, 'it's very gentle.' By this stage, the whole family had become intimately aware of my pooing (or lack thereof) predicament. The consensus was to go for it.

Within an hour I had my first small bowel motion after almost four months. I was so relieved, not just physically but emotionally. It did not even hurt. I was unscathed. I was fine. My new rectum worked! I quickly called Zak who immediately spread the good news. I would be able to come home tomorrow. I then sat down to eat a little dinner when two spoonfuls into the soup I got the urge to go again. Wow, this felt good! Repositioning myself in front of the slightly cooled bowl of soup, the urge once again returned. In fact between the hours of 6pm and 2am, it returned around 19 times!

Aside from the inconvenience of a broken night's sleep and rawness in my bottom, I am overwhelmingly grateful that my bowels are back in action and that my system has well and truly been flushed out. Goodbye old, hello new.

I couldn't hide my smile as I departed the following morning with one less bag than on check-in. Hand in hand, Danny and I excitedly left the hospital, unencumbered and feeling free.

xxxooo

Would you believe Journal 2 ends right here ... I love it, perfectly aligned with the end of that stage.

(Above: Special welcome back toilet paper that Danny found in Lithuania of all places!)

Journal Three

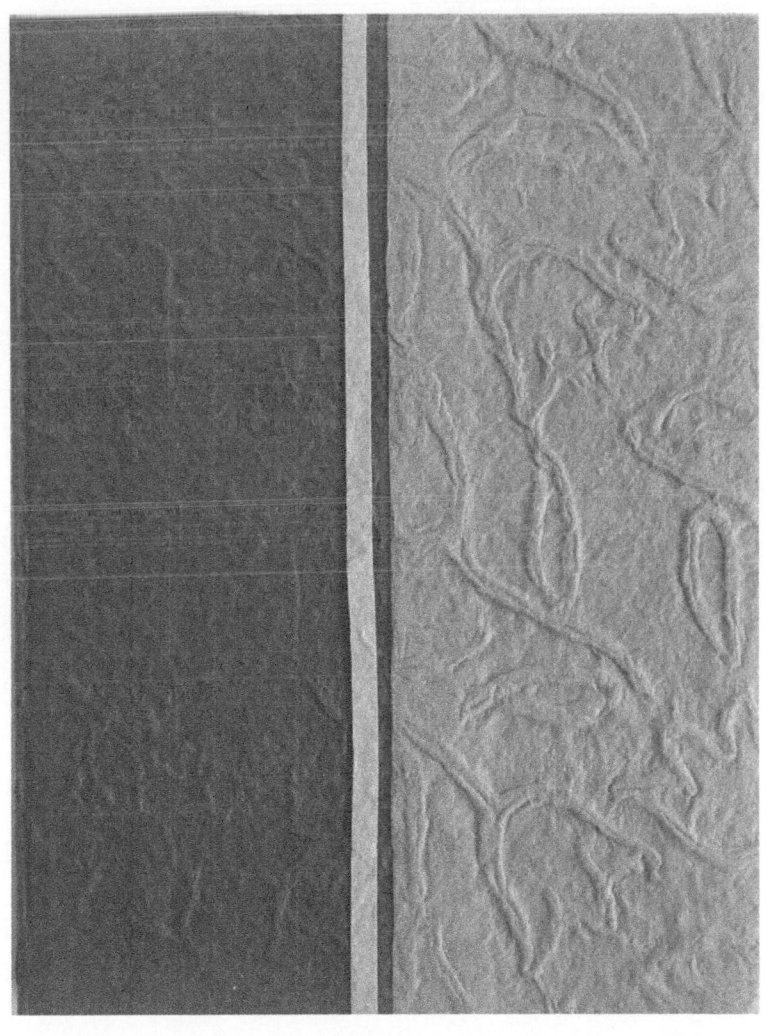

15 October 2011

Back Home (again!)

I am feeling so grateful. I am doing brilliantly. I can breathe. I'm amazed at how daily, focused, intentional breathing impacts the way I feel—relaxed, restored and repaired.

* 5 deep breaths in (I can actually breathe quite deeply, if I build it up slowly). I set an intention, for example healing in the bowel
* Hold for 5 seconds
* Exhale for 5 seconds

Ten or so minutes are truly restorative, especially when I direct my breathing to the operation site.

Mindfully I place my hands on my stomach area, forming a love heart that encircles my belly button. I begin breathing in healing words, taking purposefully deep, slow breaths. Intuitively I move the 'love heart' around to desired areas, a bit like an Ouija (or wigi) board that effortlessly glides to the vibrations of departed souls. I am at one with my breath, magically purifying and balancing my body and soul.

Healing hands

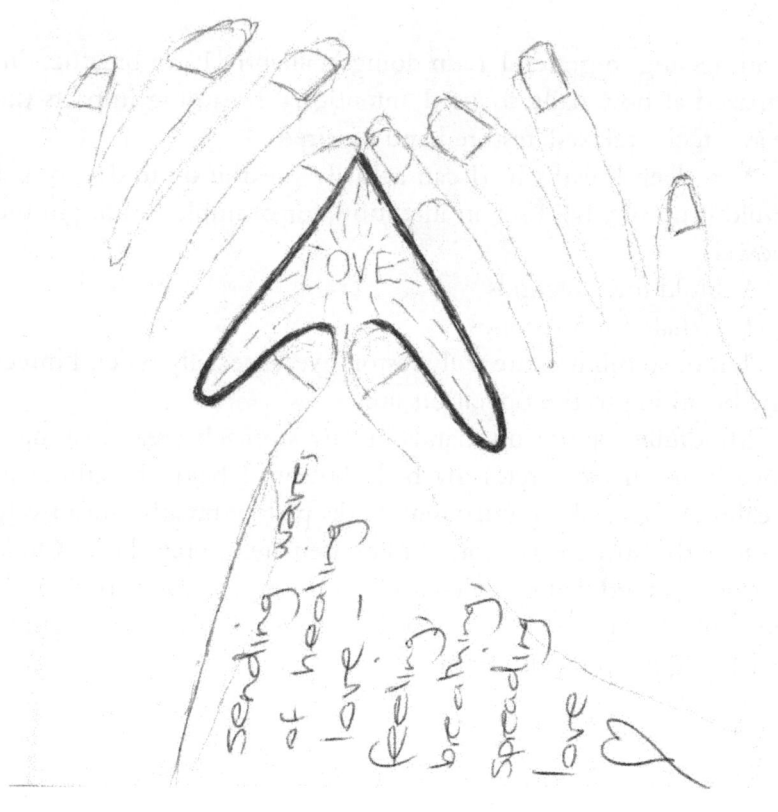

LOVE

Sending waves
of healing
pure love
feeling
breathing
spreading
love

Mindful Body Scan

This practice is great to do everyday, even if only for a moment. Regular practice will help heighten your senses, making you more attuned to how your body is feeling in the present moment. Try doing this scan from a position of acceptance and without judgment.

To begin find a comfortable spot to sit or lie so you are fully supported and relaxed.

1. Close your eyes
2. Gently ease into a more relaxed state paying attention to the natural rhythm of your breath. Notice the difference in temperature from the cool air as you inhale to the warmer air as you exhale
3. Bring awareness to your body as a whole. Notice how your body feels as it comes into contact with the cushion on the chair, the mattress or the floor. How your clothes feel as they rest on your body
4. Begin focusing your attention on different parts of your body beginning with your toes, and then slowly progress through to each foot, heel, sole, the lower and upper part of your legs, pelvis, abdomen, lower back, upper back, chest, arms down to the fingers, shoulders, neck, and then to the different parts of your face and head
5. For each part of the body linger for a moment noticing any different sensations that arise as you focus your attention. Spend a little longer directing additional love and healing in areas where there may be pain or tension
6. If you lose your attention or begin to doze off, don't worry just gently reawaken yourself with a deep breath and return your attention to the last part of body you remember focusing on
7. When you have finished this body scan practice, lie for just one more moment before placing a gentle smile of gratitude on your face in appreciation of your body's amazing conscious and unconscious functioning. Then open your eyes.

17 October 2011

Changing Roles

When illness befalls someone in a family, so much changes, yet at the same time so much stays the same. Some familial bonds strengthen, whilst others are put to the test. Over the course of a lifespan, multiple occasions arise when our static roles are hurled into chaos: from person to patient, partner to carer, child to helper and mum/partner/friend/daughter to a person in need. Same person, different needs. Some occur as part of a natural order, which in some respects can make it easier to accept, for example becoming a parent or caring for an ageing parent, but others are more random such as an unexpected illness.

During periods of change some people morph between roles seamlessly, while others offer up resistance or even become unhinged. Creatures of habit, why would we seek to change unless we have to? When you're a child why would you want to become a de facto mum or dad? Or if you're a romantic partner, being other-focused for extended periods can strain even the closest of bonds. During times of crises, a fluidity of roles is required, but I admit it can be easier said than done. It takes time, encouragement and a flexible mind to bend with the altered flow.

In my role once again as 'home-patient', I'm impatient and frustrated by many things such as the lack of ready meals in the fridge. Isn't it obvious that when someone returns from hospital meals are to be organised? I later find out assistance was offered but for the large part declined by my beloved. Hello! Excess food can always be frozen and having a choice is a great thing, especially with so many fusspots in the family. I know this has been a comparatively minor operation but still.

Moving on!

For kids, is it too much to expect an automatic shift towards greater responsibility? Unprompted, can't they at least figure out that a dirty bowl on the table (shock horror!) goes into the dishwasher? This is not a manoeuvre specifically designed for adults! It appears some things need to be pointed out and aren't built-in adaptations kicking in automatically and intuitively when the need arises. Perhaps that does not really matter, the main thing is that people respond accordingly, making an effort to be adaptive and the earlier in life this is learnt, the better. It's a necessary part of growth and evolution as human beings, honing our empathetic and adaptive skills. Stepping out of your comfort zone can also provide opportunities for personal growth and demonstrate what we need to learn the most.

Learning to communicate your expectations and needs is really important, although this often needs to be negotiated and worked at. Importantly, imparting such pearls of wisdom is not the best idea during times of heightened stress. In case you haven't realised, I am writing this for my own benefit! I was just trying to be polite.

Until my family's psychic abilities have been mastered, I know exactly what I need to learn: patience and conveying my needs calmly. I can't assume people to become a mini-mum or mini-Ros. Everyone sees things from their own perspective. One person's obvious is another's optional. Yet I believe that, at the core of human nature, people love being helpful. That's why altruism, helping others—which leads to a certain form of helping high—improves our wellbeing. The symbiotic act of giving and receiving: a blurring of the two definitions.

I am now realising it's time to shift from rant mode to acknowledging the many positive transformations that have already taken place. Thank you Zak for taking your cooking levels up at least one notch, Danny for trying your best, including shopping, schlepping, and making the arduous shift from creative dreamer to practical doer, and thank you Josh for offering to make me cups of tea and generally being as obliging as you are.

To quote one of my favourite novels *To Kill a Mockingbird,* 'You never really understand a person until you consider things from his point of view ... until you climb inside of his skin and walk around in it,' which in the instance of recovering from an operation, is thankfully not something they are able to do, nor something I would ever wish they could do. I'll be content with some general TLC, applicable for all 'under the weather' moments, and certainly wouldn't say no to extra attention and spoiling. The dog at least seems to have mastered this.

What has been the most significant role change you have experienced?

....

....

....

What was your greatest challenge during this time?

....

....

....

What was the biggest lesson you learnt about yourself?

....

....

....

Compared to other people in your family, how adaptive do you think you are?

....

....

....

18 October 2011

Holy Crap

The enormity of what I have gone through these past few months has finally hit me. That first operation ... boy was it humungous!

Having had so far led a life free of operations, I had no prior experience of what to expect. After operation numero uno, my body felt like it had been run and reversed over, time and again by a semi-trailer. This can probably explain the sheer delight and relief I felt in waking up from the second operation, breathing, moving, and even laughing a little.

Still, I would not go as far as saying, as one nurse put it to me, that in comparison it was like 'a walk in the park'. If it were a park comparison, it would be an unkempt, poorly lit, overgrown park in a rough neighbourhood. I'm so grateful to have had the harder operation first, and not the other way around, and that it was now, while I am young. I have such admiration for older and frailer people who have gone through and recovered from operations such as these. I am recalling the gastroenterologist's words when I was at the height of my deliberations saying, 'If you were my grandmother I'd suggest the lesser bowel resection but as you are a young woman with two young children I'd recommend the full bowel resection.'

What an assault on the body—a physical, emotional and mental onslaught. I have employed so much inner strength to regain my energy and physicality. How much more would someone nearly double my age need? And let's face it, the average age range for these operations is the late 50s–70s. How many would not bounce back? And if they did, how extensive would the physical and emotional toll be?

I know I will recover. I will regain strength and, in time, the trauma of what I have been through will diminish. May my future ahead be extensive and expansive, and blessed by good health.

Visualisation Exercise: The Healthy You

When you are sick for a long time, there is a risk you can almost forget what it's like to feel well and energised.

Spend some time now (and on days you crave more energy and vitality) visualising feeling well and having lots of energy. Really sense into this feeling kinaesthetically—using all your senses: smell, touch, taste, sound and sight. You don't have to spend long doing this; even just a few moments will help reprogram cellular memory and reconnect you to your healthy self.

What image comes to mind? I often imagine jogging around the park on a sunny blue-sky day, my hair blowing in the wind – such an invigorating feeling.

---

20 October 2011

Mind over (faecal) matter

All those months ago when I was agonisingly deciding which operation to choose, I remember the specialist recounting some of the longer and shorter-term outcomes of having a full bowel resection. Knowing this to be the only choice ultimately right for me, and with an already overloaded mind, I didn't pay too much attention or even fully relate to many details he imparted. I dismissed them into the worry-about-later pile. Of these were the likelihood of more frequent bowel motions, a feeling of incomplete bowel movements, unreliability of motions and possible incontinence.

To me, incontinence could only refer to weeing, certainly not pooing. I mean how disgusting! Microsoft Word does not even acknowledge 'pooing' as a real word. Upon leaving the hospital, I was told to expect irregularity and an unreliable bowel for the next few weeks.

Now I am coming to understand what the surgeon was talking about. I'm feeling very insecure and uncertain I won't involuntarily do a poo. When I'm upright the force of gravity is so strong, I immediately want to lie down if only to be on the safe side. My bum (inside and out) is like that of a newborn baby: red, raw and sore. Faecal matter passes both painfully and slowly through a shorter, patched up bowel that has not seen action for four months.

As for my rectum, although I don't look any different since the operation, it is forever altered. With my rather keen (or sick) sense of humour, I keep breaking into a smile, delighted I now have the best response for the icebreaker activity, 'Tell everyone something about yourself they would not know about you.' To which I would respond, 'I have a spanking new (no pun intended—wink) rectum.' I'll definitely have to recall this for latter use!

Aside from the warped and mildly humorous aspect, each day that passes brings more challenges for my new rectum. As soon as the urge comes, I dash to the toilet for what I anticipate to be a large motion. Instead what yields is something smaller than and of similar consistency to a garden pebble that agonisingly descends, like a razor-edged stone, millimetre-by-millimetre. At times it feels once again like I'm giving birth, but rather than a seven-pound baby, out strains a one-ounce poo accompanied by tears flowing down my cheeks.

Continuing on the rebirth theme, I am slathering myself in Sudocrem, last used for the boys nappy rash, as confirmed by the decade-old expiration date. Of course I know these are early days, but toilet training is not something I'd ever envisaged revisiting for myself. I am actively retraining my brain, nervous system and bowel to understand which signals to pay attention to: when to dash to the loo, when to hold it in, when it's a fart as opposed to a poo and when it's safe to leave the close proximity of a toilet.

How grateful I am to be young, have good muscle tone, a strong pelvic floor and to be openly prepared to challenge my body's current limitations, putting in place some serious mind training.

I will control my bowel and my rectum, not the other way around. In time, order will be restored and going to the toilet will revert to being just another part of my daily routine. For now I need to accept that time, as well as strengthening my mind-body connection are important parts of healing. How I feel today is not how I will feel tomorrow. On more challenging days I will delight in closing my eyes knowing tomorrow will always bring a fresh start brimming with new possibilities. I will celebrate small milestones. I will get stronger and soon my new rectum will bear a 'P' plate instead of its current 'L'.

X

Has there been a time in your life you actively engaged your mind-body connection to enhance healing?

....

....

....

What did you do? For example affirmations, yoga, tai chi?

....

....

....

Outline a mind-body practice you can do right now to promote healing and wellbeing?

....

....

....

22 October 2011

How to respond to 'How are you?'

Ten plus days post-op and almost one week home, I am wondering how to respond to the question 'How are you?' Saying I am doing really well paints an image in people's minds that I am fine, and more or less recovered. I have become the penultimate white liar, even to myself. I don't like outwardly complaining. I want to be positive, aware of the importance of a positive mindset for healing. Each time I speak the harsh truth it feels like I'm admonishing myself.

As a result of downplaying how I'm really feeling, meals drops and phone calls enquiring about my welfare are now sporadic. Of the calls I do receive they exemplify a normal tone, for example, 'Do you want to go for a walk?' 'Do you want to have coffee?' as opposed to 'How are you feeling today?'

I am left wondering how to best respond to this seemingly common question. The reality of having a younger set of friends, late 30s to early 50s, is that on the whole and thankfully they can't fully relate to ill health, beyond a bad bout of flu, broken bones or hormonal issues. Adding to this is the unfortunate location of the area of my operation itself and the fact that the subsequent discomforts pertain to poo. I can't say there are too many people I could or would want to give a blow-by-blow account of all things bowel or faecal. If I could, then they would hear about the labour of my first week of toilet training, the all-consuming, searing pain of feeling parts of my bowel I never even knew existed, using both elbows to prop up my weary head after long stretches of hopeful waiting on the loo—so long that my hands temporarily etch impressions into my cheeks. I too could not have envisaged what life with a new rectum would be like, so I really can't expect others to understand the enormity of what I am currently undergoing.

On top of this comes my frustration at people's (and society's) attitude to poo-related matters or toileting behaviour outside of the toddler set. They either become awkwardly silent and uncomfortable, verging on embarrassed, or bemused in an almost infantile way complete with sniggering and guffawing. Now that ain't the type of laughter I like! I would imagine other people who have had removal or replacement of other sensitive body parts might feel similarly. Some body parts are definitely easier to talk about than others. I doubt many people would give an awkward thought to discussing the replacement of a finger or toe!

For the most part I imagine most people wouldn't give it too much thought, assuming it's like your system normalising after a bad bout of gastro. How could anyone imagine how painful bowel refunctioning would be after a lengthy dormancy? Muscles withered, contracted and lying dormant, only to be rudely awakened, not to normal functioning—although that would be challenging enough—but to a whole new set of rules. This system of mine has not been restored to its original 'factory' settings. Instead, more than 20cm of the original hardware inclusive of the anal pouch has been removed and replaced with a new, man-made, custom-designed pouch which, as extraordinary as it sounds and regardless of the skilled hands of my surgeon, is devoid of the miraculous qualities of our blessed, birth-given, perfect body.

I'm not returning to normal, because the goal posts of normalcy have forever been removed. Soon, all being well, my brain and bowel will readjust and any previous standard will become a blurry haze, replaced by a new normal and an inability to recall it ever being different. In the meantime I am navigating the unknown. My brain is attempting to teach itself a new language. A lot of healing still needs to be done. I want the new normal to be better than the previous one. I'm acknowledging my nervous system's grumbling, 'What the hell?' I need to continue working at creating a well-functioning digestive and excretory system.

I now have a new level of understanding as to why there is a four-week recovery period after the bowel reconnection.

I have decided the following. When people ask how I am, I don't need to give them a detailed and full account of what has been going on day-by-day, hour-by-hour. Instead I'll keep it general saying, 'I'm doing really well, all things considered' and possibly add something about the process of readjustment. If it feels appropriate I may divulge more but I want my inner conscious and unconscious mind to hear how well I am doing to encourage and optimise healing. And I don't like being a liar.

X X

How do you respond to 'How are you?' when you've got something big going on and you don't feel great? (Marathon vs. a few days under the weather)

....

....

....

How does it make you feel when you respond honestly (warts and all) versus non-specific and generalised language e.g. I'm doing OK, or fine. Consider the response best suited to you.

....

....

....

24 October 2011

A bug or a blessing?

One of my closest friends came around this week with a lovingly prepared meal. She stayed a while distracting me from my discomfort and we parted sharing a long embrace.

Two days later in trepidation she called, divulging she had come down with one of the worst gastro bugs she had ever had and wanted to make sure I was OK. I could hear her relief when I relayed I was fine. She conveyed the lengths to which she had gone with food preparation, even donning disposable gloves, something she had taken to doing when cooking for her terminally ill mother and a measure I admit I would not have taken myself. I thanked her for all her efforts and told her how much we all appreciated her tasty food, before once again reassuring her I felt absolutely fine.

I didn't really give it another thought until, fast-forward 24 hours, growing nausea, a racing heart and that sinking feeling let me know it was only a matter of time before the gastro bug would latch onto my insides. The 'what ifs' lost no time forming in my mind. How would I cope? How much pain would I be in when the vomiting started? In fact, I had already moved beyond the 'if' to the 'when'.

I hoped I would be spared these agonies and the bug would pass from my system without wreaking too much devastation. Willing the rising nausea away, with heavy eyes, I prayed for sound sleep. Miraculously, the night passed without too much drama and the next morning I praised myself on how hard I had worked to quell the virus. Wow, I really must be strong, I coped so well. The 'I am strong', 'I am healthy and well' affirmations worked so well. Still light-headed I enjoyed a restful day delighted that all the contents of my scarred bowel remained within.

A couple days passed and with it went my post-op energy, leaching from my system like sap from a damaged branch, until I could no longer raise my head from the pillow. I recalled the words of my oncology psychologist that sometimes you just need a 'pyjama day'. Legs like jelly, head like a dead weight, the whole day passed sluggishly, only moving to get a drink, go to the toilet or have another horizontal lying experience on a different couch or bed. Surely I'll feel better by tomorrow?

The next day arrived and I was filled with hope that my rest would have paid off and my energy levels would be restored. One step out of bed quickly established this was not the case. I was alerted to the gentle tingling sensation in the right side of my face confirming the awakening of my stress-response, a cold sore virus, from dormancy. I recalled how my healthy friend told me she had never been sicker in her life. I also remembered how in the past my naturopath had complimented my body for its strong reactions—a sign of a healthy response system—despite how at odds it was with my present feelings. At times I even wondered if this was a clever strategy she employed to make me feel better about my ridiculously over-sensitive system. But maybe she was right. My overloaded and weakened immune system couldn't wage this war or prevent this bug from setting foot in my body.

Talking to friends about my gastro bug highlighted people's different worldviews. I was struck at how many viewed it as bad luck, something terrible, a real setback. Of course I would have preferred not to get this bug, but I genuinely and naturally felt the positive flip side; and in any case, there wasn't much I could do about it. It just was. Making peace helped strip away some of my frustration. I offered less resistance and created more space for healing. Just as the food was delivered with love, so too was the virus. Its raison d'être was to slow me down, stop me in my tracks and allow my body to heal from this operation. I had already started accelerating, pushing myself too much and expecting far too much from myself.

As I write, a Talmudic tale about perspective keeps coming to mind that goes something like this:

Once there was a farmer who had only one horse, and one day the horse ran away. The neighbours came to console him over his terrible loss. The farmer said, 'It's neither good nor bad, it is.'

A month later, the horse returned home, this time bringing with her two beautiful wild horses. The neighbours were happy for the farmer's good fortune. Such lovely strong horses! The farmer said, 'It's neither good nor bad, it is.'

One day while riding one of the wild horses, the farmer's son was thrown and broke his leg. All the neighbours were very distressed. Such bad luck! The farmer said, 'It's neither good nor bad, it is.'

Then a war came, and every able-bodied man was conscripted and sent into battle. Only the farmer's son, because he had a broken leg, remained. The neighbours congratulated the farmer. 'It's neither good nor bad, it is,' said the farmer.

The reality is we can never really fully understand the universal truth or purpose behind anything. We only understand it from our earthly perspective. I also have a newfound appreciation for my friend and the lengths she went to ensure the meal's safeness and freshness! She hadn't factored in the hug but why should she have? She had been feeling fine the afternoon she visited.

Have you ever had an illness or a perceived bad thing happen, only to learn later that it was a blessing in disguise? If you're still struggling to find the blessing, consider some of the positive outcomes of this 'negative' event?

....

....

....

1 November 2011

Scheduling 'downtime'

Remaining positive, day after day, when you're feeling lousy takes its toll and I am quite fed up. Like a pendulum my mind vacillates between the 'it's neither good nor bad, it is' perspective with no judgment and the 'woe is me' castigating mode.

Daytime TV sucks and I don't have the headspace to write or energy to read. Quickly I descend into the depths of despair consumed by the constant sight of blood in my stools, the discomfort, and the uncertainty of my bowel motions. What's wrong with me? Why can't I shake this lethargy? I'm feeling the need to call the surgeon to calm my mind and allay any fears. I think I may need blood tests and an examination, but it's Sunday and a long weekend for the holy Cup Day horse race, so I am in mixed minds about disturbing him. After a chat with my brother I hesitatingly page him but he is on leave, and I'm redirected to another specialist, the head of the hospital colorectal group. Not long passes before he returns my call and I relay my symptoms. He isn't overly concerned but tells me to call him if I start feeling worse.

Skip ahead 24 hours and I do feel worse. I really did not think I would, but I have come to realise that feeling better is not something I can just will to happen, or expect it to, no matter how positive I am.

Another call and I'm back at the hospital for a rectal examination and blood tests. My anxiety levels go down as he assures me that all is basically within the realms of normalcy on the physical level. Perhaps my setback was due to the virus? The specialist asks for one word to describe how I feel and I respond 'depleted'. What I really want to say is 'fucking lousy', but that's two.

More days pass flopping from bed to couch to bed to floor, mindlessly channel-flicking and becoming increasingly frustrated. My sleep has been restless, characterised by vivid dreams and restless, twitching muscles aching to exercise. There has been none of that these past few weeks.

I'm so tired and the words from Year 12 French, 'Je suis fatiguée,' constantly come to mind, amusing me as I can't remember any other French phrases! I keep thinking I should be feeling better. I'm sure other people would be feeling better by now. I'm dangerously close to succumbing to the affliction of comparison-itis. I don't like moaning and whinging to friends or family but I have to do something about all this pent up frustration.

A book I have begun flicking through about anxiety in children advocates setting aside 15 minutes of your day to voice your worries and concerns. So with this advice fresh in my mind I decide to have a whinge/complaint session. I really need to. I've had enough. I want to feel well with as little effort as possible and it has just not been happening at the speed I desire. 'It takes so much strength to be strong' seems to be my new motto but I'm just not feeling that strong.

Heeding the book's advice I decide to indulge in whinge time, to get it out of my system. Out loud I unfurl all the negative talk occupying my mind, and it feels great. This process feels both heavy and light: heavy is the load of negativity that exits and light the sense of being that enters. Innately I know when I have said enough, and slowly and cautiously I pull in the reigns; all this negativity is over-saturating and actually makes me feel physically ill with its toxic venom as it passes in, and then out of my system. It's really quite overpowering.

I take a few deep breaths in and regain composure. Another few deep breaths in and out. I start considering all the blessings in my life and all that I'm grateful for. At first it feels like I am pedalling uphill as I nudge myself to persevere with positive talk. Gradually I no longer need to force myself as genuine and effortless positivity flows in and throughout me. The darkness embodied in all that negative expression has vanished.

I am freer, unencumbered, even though nothing physically has really changed—just my mindset. I now know I will be better company not only to others but also to myself. After all I do have to live with me! Nobody likes negativity but at times we all succumb to its power. When you're feeling great with no present challenges, it's so much easier being upbeat. The trick is to harness a positive outlook when you are drained, fatigued, downhearted or frustrated. When unchecked, these feelings too easily dominate over hope and vitality.

I love this idea of scheduling down time, in order to reap up time. It is so important to acknowledge the full spectrum of emotions, to have an active dialogue in order to reach equilibrium. Just make sure you allocate a time boundary that will allow enough minutes to rid your system of negativity. Then welcome back positive talk. You don't want to get lost wallowing.

Think of a negative thought stored inside you.

....

....

....

Allow some time to dump it from your system, either through drawing, writing or talking it out.

Once you're done, regain composure, perhaps by taking a few deep breaths in and then out. Initially you may feel a little churned up by this process, but in time you will feel better for it.

7 November 2011

Sick and tired of feeling sick and tired

All I can think about is how exhausted I am. Even with focused breathing exercises and power naps (they sure don't feel like 'power' naps), I lapse into 'tired language'. If Zak or anyone else asks me to do something I automatically respond, 'I am too tired.' The same goes for when I am asked to go for a walk, and before I know it my whole day is filled with vocalised and silent renditions of 'I'm tired.'

Yesterday I caught myself mid fatigue thought realising this line of thinking had become my default. Metaphorically I slapped my butt, reminding myself I needed to embrace a more positive orientation and say things like, 'I love having lots of energy,' 'I love feeling vitality,' etc. So over the course of the next 36 hours that's exactly what I did. Time and again as my thought patterns erred towards the fatigue/frustration arrow, I steered them in a positive direction with a new set of affirmations: 'I love having lots of energy,' 'It makes me feel wonderful,' 'My body is a wonderful healer.'

In some ways, not acknowledging my fatigue felt a little fraudulent, but a negative disposition has neither enhanced my mood nor brought a skip to my stride. If there was some way to gauge how long I would be feeling like this, then I could at least psych myself up for that period of time. It is like when you're in between jobs and fail to be as productive as you could or fully enjoy life during that period as the uncertain timing of future employment cues apathy, not action.

I know, not even deep down but closer to the surface, it is just a matter of time. I've been in the red enough times before to know after a spell of despondency the fog lifts and life returns to normal.

I consider the vast reserves of mental energy required for people with less hope: people with terminal illnesses or life-long disabilities for whom finite becomes infinite, for whom the future links so inextricably to present circumstances and hope is beyond grasp.

I hope it's not just wishful thinking but I'm feeling a wisp of energy, like a ragged patch of grassy green emerging from a snowy field. There is hope; I just have to wait for the thaw to spread. I don't know how much I can attribute this to a conscious shift in attitude, but something has changed and I feel the best I have in ages. Perhaps it was the mindful walk I took around the park, matching my paces with conscious breaths. It was wonderful. No dog, just my thoughts and myself together in nature. What a simple, enjoyable and effective way to orient towards a more positive outlook.

Have you ever been for a mindful walk? It really is a wonderful way to become present and mindful of our body, thoughts and breath.

Mindful Walking Exercise (10 - 15 minutes)

Time to allocate some you-time, free of any apendages (human or pet).

You can either do this mindful walking practice inside or outside. If you are doing it inside or on a freshly manicured lawn, consider removing your shoes for added grounding and sensual benefits.

First just spend a moment standing in stillness, noticing how the soles of your shoes or feet feel as they connect to the floor or ground. Take a couple of deep breaths in and then out. Look around, particularly if you are outside in nature and become aware of your surroundings. Hone your senses into any sounds, sights, smells or other sensations that capture your attention. Try and let go of any intrusive thoughts or emotions. Notice how your arms fall by your sides and how your breath moves in and out of your body. You don't need to change anything, just let it be.

Become aware of your legs and your feet planted firmly on the ground, then lift your right foot up, moving it forward, and place it back down. Mindfully shift the weight from your right leg to your left leg, lifting your left foot up, moving it forward, and then placing it back on the ground. This is what mindful walking is all about, repeating this process, over and over again and being aware of any bodily sensations: the soles of your feet, your legs, your arms as they sway back and forward. You are now walking in a state of awareness, one step at a time.

If you are doing this practice inside, at some point you will need to turn. Do so while maintaining the flow of mindfulness and begin walking back to where you started, one step at a time, at a rhythm that suits you. Or perhaps you can walk in a circle (just don't get dizzy!)

Notice any thoughts that arise and let them be, returning your focus to the sensation of walking. Lifting, moving, placing.

Notice your breath. Does the rhythm match your pace of walking? Why not add rhythmic breathing to your walking? Breathe in for a count of 5 as you walk 5 paces and then exhale for a count of 5 as you walk 5 paces and repeat for some time. If counting to 5 is too long to maintain, begin by breathing up to 3 counts and then out for another 3. In time you can build up to longer breaths. You can slow down your counting to encourage slower walking or quicken it, alternating walking slowly for a period of time (or around the room) and then more quickly. This combines rhythmic breathing with rhythmic walking and is a great way to become fully present.

Practice walking mindfully for a few moments (with or without counting). Notice how your whole body interplays with breath, pace and movement, coordinating and connecting body, mind and spirit.

Spend a moment noticing the stillness when you stop walking.

You have just discovered a whole new way of walking.

13 November 2011

My hidden laughter self

The notion of staying positive in the face of adversity came closer to home today whilst catching up with my phone buddy: a lovely lady referred via the sister of a good friend who'd had the same operation as me, about six months before mine, while just a few months younger than me, at 42. She is a wonderful source of inspiration and hope, especially as she has emerged on the other side in overall good health.

I've adopted her gem of advice: hoola hooping one way and then another to relieve trapped wind which I now do on an almost daily basis. It really helps! Living in central NSW, our friendship has been confined to the telephone. In one of our previous lengthy and heartfelt conversations she remarked how much happier she now felt and how her whole life view had changed. Like me, she has lost the taste for small talk. Our phone conversations always leave me uplifted, relieved, and filled with hope. I marvel at how close I feel to someone I have never met and with whom I've only shared a mere three conversations.

In our last chat she told me she was having further genetic testing conducted on the polyp. I too had these tests done and thankfully was given the all-clear. It had been a while since I had heard from her and I was excited to let her know I'd had the bowel reconnection. As soon as I heard her voice on the other end of the phone, I knew something was not right. She relayed the genetic testing revealed a gene that predisposed her to a range of cancers, most specifically ovarian and uterine. My heart sank as she told me she was in the midst of psyching herself up for further surgery: a hysterectomy in the short term and down the track, the removal of her ovaries.

This was someone with no genetic history of cancer and two young children. The looming reality of what lay ahead had, unsurprisingly, weathered her optimism, and she confided that she was not coping very well, snapping at her kids and not laughing anymore.

On the tip of my tongue were the words I had wanted to tell her in earlier conversations; I was a laughter wellness therapist. But for whatever reason, I held back. Now it just seemed inappropriate. I told her it was not at all surprising she did not feel like laughing with all the heavily laden decisions she had to make. Huge decisions that, no matter how positive you are, you can't just magic away. With toned down authority, I told her how important it was to spend time with people who make you feel good, to try and put a smile on your face at the beginning and end of each day, even if it's the last thing you feel like doing, and to watch some comedy.

I was on the verge of telling her that perhaps I could help bring some laughter back into her life, but it did not feel like the right time or right conversation. To this day I can't really explain why I held back from exposing my laughter side. One menacing thought was that if laughter was such good medicine, then as a laughter and health promotion practitioner (albeit part time) why did I get sick in the first place? This wasn't the first time I'd suppressed that thought, and it deeply troubled me.

I often feel uncomfortable explaining to new clients, particularly those with chronic health issues, how laughter can help, how therapeutic it really is. The last thing you want to convey is that you're making light of someone's situation, suggesting they just 'laugh it off'. Embracing a 'laughter mentality' is complex and hard to grasp at the best of times; but especially when you're ensconced by fear and darkness.

I liken laughter to a stream of light that can filter through any darkened space. It just needs a crack to enter, and then, like magic, it effortlessly penetrates and overshadows the darkness.

Laughter (like a beam of light)

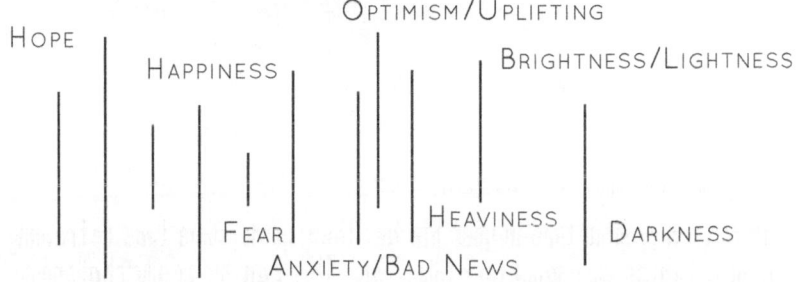

All I wanted was to give her hope, but there's nothing worse than false hope and I certainly didn't want to share that. I told her I thought she would be alright, with an unspoken mutual understanding that this 'alright' would in all probability be far removed from the type of 'alright' we aspire to be.

It's so easy maintaining and embracing hope when future prospects are rosy. In her case, hopefully, the knowledge of having this particular gene will maximise a healthy, cancer-free future, but I keep thinking what I am sure she was also thinking, 'at what cost?'. Surgery to remove one thing, followed by the scheduling to remove something else—a path beset by shadows.

I feel so blessed knowing that all being well I rid my body of any traces of cancer, and I can breathe in the knowledge that I am free of any lingering cancerous cells or mutation potential. It does not diminish how frustrated I feel at the moment—or the reality of the, at times, hellish recovery over the past six months—but that's it: a finite period that will conclude a challenging chapter in my life. As for my phone pal, she's still on the conveyer belt of medical interventions, and whilst surgery is the best solution in many regards, no surgery comes easily or without unintended consequences, and a huge physical and emotional toll.

My hope for her is that love and laughter will bolster her through this challenging period. Living without laughter is like extinguishing hope, depleting your whole self of the very stuff that can miraculously make even the worst situation feel a little bit little lighter and brighter.

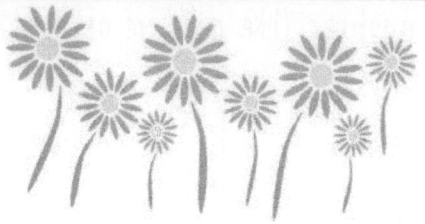

LEARNING TO LAUGH AT YOUR PAIN

Think of a painful time in your life and then spend some time reframing it in a lighter and laughter-filled way. This can be really challenging, but truly worthwhile. It will help free your brain of some of the pain and trauma you have been carrying around with you (consciously and/ or unconsciously), helping to change the way it remembers this episode.

....
....
....
....
....

meditation

one small shift:
from medication
to meditation ♡

22 November 2011

Doin' Time: the long haul

This morning marks six weeks post-op. The official recovery time, the time when the skip in my stride should have returned, and zest and energy re-embedded into my whole self.

Initially I was told a three to five week recovery, but with the irregular bleeding the surgeon said, 'No, we really mean six weeks.' I can't help but feel a little disappointed that the goal posts signifying the end of the 'official' recovery period are still out of reach.

My emotional self is deflated. It's not that I consider myself to be a healing failure, quite the contrary. In a bizarre way I have been convincing myself my longer recovery is because I am such an amazingly thorough healer. You see you can convince yourself of anything really! Even if bordering on delusional, this new way of thinking helps quell my mounting frustration.

It's one thing to accept the allotted recovery time, but another when it crosses into overtime. Frustration mounts, patience wanes, other people's patience wanes and for many bystanders, interest in the reluctant patient is entirely lost. Like a domino effect all these things can impact on recovery length and patient experience. I sometimes feel like shouting, 'Hello, I'm still here,' because after a while many people make the assumption that, 'She had that operation ages ago, she must be fine.' I do not mean this as a judgment but rather as an acknowledgement that each person's views is based on their own life experience.

As for my tireless husband and family, my being under the weather has regretfully been the norm for patches over these past decades—a perfect model of good health? Ironically, the time I received the most outward and ongoing sympathy (minus the bowel resection) was when I broke my foot. The cast served as an outward reminder of my affliction, galvanizing much higher levels of sympathy and concern than I'd ever experienced with other invisible afflictions e.g. chronic fatigue syndrome. Minus the break itself, I felt absolutely fine. Isn't that funny?

I feel the need for some more affirmations:

I know it's only a matter of time before I feel well

It's OK that it's taking a little longer to recover (I've never exactly been 'normal')

In small ways I am already feeling better

Think of a challenging time you were going through (emotional/physical/spiritual)

....

....

....

Were your support networks there for the long haul?

....

....

....

If they weren't there in the way you would have hoped, if in the future need arises, how can you ensure better support?

....

....

....

The Friendship Mosaic

My rather lengthy recovery has provided much time for contemplation: a valuable gift that for many would be a luxury. Times of crisis can be great opportunities to reflect on friendships; you certainly learn who your true friends are. I have begun compiling a friendship classification list.

Lifeline (life-long) friends

These friendships are more valuable than the rarest gem, cultivated over many years, shared life experiences or united by a common fence. These are friends who check in on your physical and emotional wellbeing on a regular basis and accompany you, hand in hand, through the bumps and lumps of life, and whose empathy is second to none. Their warmth and brimming love fills you with an inner glow that spills into your spirit. These friendships are endearing and enduring, the most treasured of all, and if things were in reverse, you'd do exactly the same. It's akin to the unconditional love you offer your children, or other close family members. You don't need many of these friendships. Even one means you are indeed blessed.

To my life-line friends: thank you for allowing me to freely whinge, moan, complain, share victories, minor and major accomplishments; for schlepping, for the constancy and consistency of your calls, and for not keeping a tally of who initiated the calls; for the thoughtful gifts, shopping, cooking, feeding us—the list goes on. Most of all though, thank you for just being there.

Sideline friends

These are friends you think will be around for the long haul of an illness and recovery, no matter how extended this may be; yet it transpires this is one marathon they watch from the sidelines, never participating in a meaningful or ongoing way. These friendships are short on stamina, bowing out well before the sweat forms. Perhaps chronic illness has skipped their path thus far, so they're lacking in the empathy department or they're simply consumed by their own competing demands and priorities. They just vanish, checking in occasionally to hear what they want to hear: that everything is fine and dandy. A coffee friendship where if one partner (i.e. me) does not initiate to meet up, alternate plans are simply not made. Soon the friendship drifts to stalemate, with hurt feelings on one side and oblivion on the other.

Of course, everyone has their own life to lead and it's everyone's prerogative how they choose to spend their time and energy. I am not disappointed per se with all these 'side-line' friendships, but I now realise my expectations were not in line with the true nature of the friendship.

In the silence of the night, alone with my thoughts, it is these friendships that gnaw at my calm. I debate whether I should just end the standoff by texting or calling, to confront them, not in a conflictive sense, more subtly, like dropping a line into a conversation, such as, 'This recovery has been much more challenging than I had expected, especially with the irregular bleeding and bout of nasty viruses.' These words may not be enough to elevate the friendship to its original status, but might secure a belated empathic response and quell my feelings of disappointment and disenchantment. But my stubborn spirit dictates 'the order' is wrong. I should not be the one to reach out to them; it should be the other way around. I am struck at how petty this seems, but as someone who has been brought up to do the 'right thing', I consistently find it hard to believe other people do not share these same values.

Inwardly I know the best thing for my own wellbeing would be to actively re-harness control and let go of any frustration and negative judgment, and focus on all the love I do have. Then it strikes me. Perhaps I'm being hypocritical, too hasty in my judgment. I don't know what has been going on in their life and maybe I haven't been there for them! For myself I need to accept that, for whatever reason, these friendships have not fully met my expectations in this present moment and without judgment.

The friend who doesn't know what to say, so remains silent

This is the friend who wants to be there for you, but is so disquieted by the cancer diagnosis, shies away. Supremely conscious of saying the wrong thing, a time lapse ensues between learning of your diagnosis and any subsequent conversation. Skirting around the 'C' issue you wonder whether perhaps your situation triggered their mortality switch to fire. Quick to judge, initially I branded their seeming inaction as a flaw rather than for what it really was; deep concern for my welfare mixed in with a hint of self-preservation. Their silence masked the unvocalised track: 'I really want to be there for you and say what you want to hear, but I just don't know what to say or do. This whole situation has really freaked me out.' Then all too soon, in an effort to make up for lost time they're compensating by doing anything for you – cooking, shopping or collecting children.

Out of the woodwork friends

These friends come out of the woodwork (and then disappear as mysteriously as they reappeared). These are friends that once played a significant role in your life who hear of your diagnosis and are the first on the phone, even the first to send flowers, deliver food and so on. They are old friendships, with a shared sense of concern and solidarity. It's so good to have these friends back in your life. Sentiment is rekindled and for a short moment you wonder what it would be like if once again they were in your life. Yet beyond this current illness you know there is insufficient shared potential in the present to progress the friendship into the future. There are no real expectations on these aged friendships, but any offerings are ever so sweet. This reconnection makes you warm on the inside, but is transitory like a wisp of smoke dissipating into the air.

The catastrophiser

Naturally these friends have your best interest at heart. I do appreciate their concern; I just don't want to drown in it. The exclamations infused with fear, 'Oh no, that's just so terrible'. It's not that I want conversations steeped in denial or wrapped up in naive positivity, but I don't need doses of angst. I want and need friends that make me feel better within myself, not highlight new concerns I had not even thought of. Thankfully this has not been a significant issue. At the whiff of a catastophiser I have deftly navigated conversations to subjects of far greater concern, such as Melbourne's weather!

Acquaintances (cyber and local)

These are people who hear about your current situation and touch base in some manner: a quick call, text or voicemail message, email or Facebook message. Those friends hover in cyber space or on the other side of the world. First contacts are rarely followed by any subsequent lengthy exchanges or face-to-face conversations, but it doesn't matter. It's lovely they took the time in the first instance to check in on my wellbeing and convey their best wishes.

The perfectionist friend

This is the type of friendship I have the most difficulty understanding: the one that promises all but delivers nothing. The friend who feels a text message or phone call is inadequate; only a face-to-face visit is appropriate. Yet owing to a whole host of reasons, this never happens. This friend is a perfectionist, who, rather than accepting the reality of our limited time, gradually distances themselves to prevent further embarrassment of being a self-perceived 'failed' friend. Ironically what they fail to understand is I would graciously and gratefully accept a less-than-perfect embodiment of friendship.

Friendships are like a waltz; if you don't both sashay in the same direction, you drift apart, no matter how committed one of the partners may be.

The new friend

Then there's the new friend, the one who suddenly appears when you need it the most; the unexpected, unscheduled person who lights up your life and makes it hard to imagine how it was before they turned up. We have that with one of our new neighbours: nothing is too much and their support to me personally and to our family is boundless.

The type of friend I think I am

So having put on my critical friendship hat, it's time to consider what type of friend I think I am. I'm hoping it will help me understand why at certain times, I've felt let down or disappointed. I know in part it is because I impose my friendship blueprint (values and expectations) on others. Sometimes I wonder how this blueprint can be so different; especially in friendships I hold so dearly and would do anything for. I mean, don't we choose our friends based on shared values?

So now a list of values I hold dear, and mirror the type of friend I think (hope) I am:
- Caring
- Nurturing
- Concerned (perhaps at times over-concerned)
- Fun (ny)
- Loving
- Empathetic
- A good listener
- Sympathetic

How I maintain my friendships:
- Phone calls
- Text message, checking in and checking up
- Emojis, yes some may think it's a copout, but I love them and at times it's all that's required
- Emails (mainly overseas)
- Facebook

- Walks
- Coffee/tea
- Outings
- Visits

If someone is sick or going through a hard time, and if for whatever reason I can't visit, I text or pick up the phone, even just for a brief moment and say, 'Hey, I am thinking of you.' I would let them know I am there for them and not just telepathically! How does it help if they don't know you're thinking about them?

I have to accept everyone expresses their love for their friends in different ways. Friendships evolve over time for a number of reasons to do with stages of life (single, with kids, etc.), physical proximity or partner incompatibility. We can't be too rigid in our assessment. Just because they wane at one time doesn't mean they won't assume renewed importance at a later date. Friendships are like waves in an ocean. You can't take more than is on offer, or give more than received. What you give, give freely and from a standpoint of love. That's the friendship flow.

It's also really important to understand that friendships can fulfil different roles; each friend can provide a different type of support and company. It makes sense to figure out who to turn to depending on what kind of connection you seek. There's no point going to someone for sympathy if they're not the sympathetic kind, just like there's no point going to someone for business advice if they're less savvy in this field than you are.

Be the type of friend you want to be; not the type others expect you to be or feel you should be. Let your sense of authentic truth guide your approach to friendship. Open your heart, and not just to those in need. When the channels of love are open, you shall not be wanting. Love breeds love, the soul food of friendships and relationships. Let your friendships serve as a model for others. Be a leading light.

When you can, relinquish negative aspects of friendships or negative and toxic friends. Release the hurt, disappointment and mismatched expectations. If you're not getting return on your investment, sometimes you have to know when to let go. Let it go. Every friendship serves a purpose. Be grateful for what you once had, for what you have now and for what you know you will have in the future.

A word of gratitude to all my friends

My deepest thanks go to all of my friends in your many shapes and forms. You have sustained me through moments of darkness and despair, joy and light. For all my friendships, even if only for a brief moment in time, you were there for a reason and made a difference. And to those few enduring priceless friendships, my chosen family, I offer my friendship as a statement of heartfelt gratitude to you. Thank you for everything.

X

What type of friend are you?

....
....
....

What do you expect from a friendship?

....
....
....

What do you view as the most important virtues of a friendship?

....
....
....

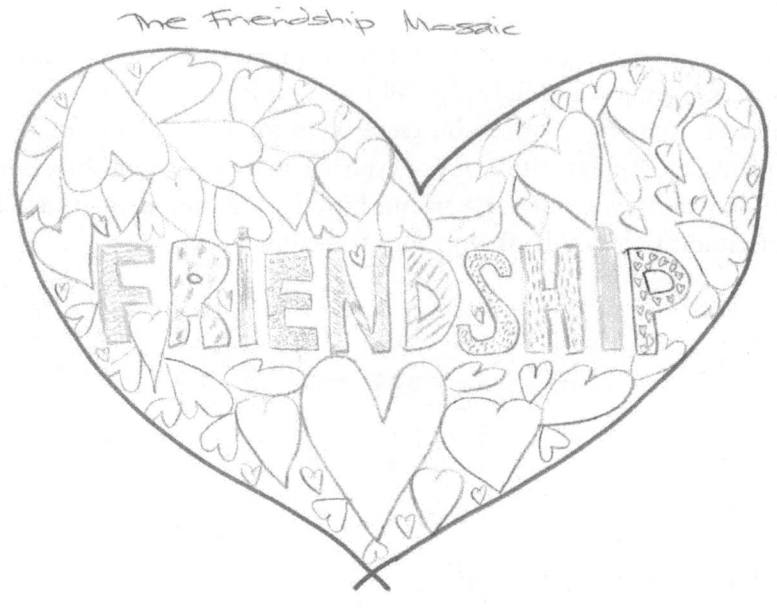

(Above: The Friendship Mosaic - Some are specks, some are chunks, some larger and some smaller; yet all are significant and together form the full mosaic.)

30 November 2011

I am more than the sum of my parts!

Seven weeks post-op and the bleeding still hasn't stopped. It wanes, almost disappears, then starts to trickle and once again flow. I am depleted and frustrated and am beginning to question if I'll be OK to go to Israel. Anxiety levels peak once again in the wee hours of the morning, prompting a call to the specialist. I need to find out what is going on and am granted an immediate appointment.

Blood tests are ordered to check blood count and I'm told that if I want to get the ever-present nausea and fatigue investigated I will need two separate referrals: one to a general physician and the other to a gastroenterologist.

The colorectal specialist doesn't seem to have any explanation as to what's going on. A disciple of modern medicine, his sole focus was on the bleeding, which is of course why I was in his examination room, but in my current state, it felt myopic. I wanted an answer for all my concerns. The physical examination was aborted, too unbearably painful.

Blood counts came back low, matching my mood. I have been so strong throughout this whole process, yet now I'm struggling to stay strong and positive. I want my strength back. I crave for it to return, for the bleeding to stop and for life to return to normal (or better than normal). I'm sick of checking the toilet bowl for traces of blood and examining the toilet paper for blood. Enough is enough. Isn't it?

Another consultation with the specialist. In my head I'm in a similar space to where I was months ago: confused, a little scared and questioning why this is happening to me. Yet another colonoscopy is discussed, but later dismissed as deemed too risky. It has only been seven weeks since the last operation and joins may not be strong enough yet to bear such an intrusion.

So a flexible sigmoidoscopy to examine the rectum and the lower colon is booked, requiring only a very light general anaesthetic, for the very next day. If nothing else I marvel at the expansion of my gastrointestinal vocabulary. I hope this will provide the (simple) answer we are looking for, but am forewarned that if anything is found and needs to be attended to, it will have to wait for another time.

I am feeling particularly low, lonely and isolated. The advantage of the procedure being booked for the next day is that I don't have too much time to get bogged down in my thoughts, although that doesn't prevent the fearful ones from leaping in and consuming me. I'm just grateful I don't have to prepare for a colonoscopy!

On our way to the hospital the next morning, Danny and I had run out of conversation. Our moods were similarly sombre. The British comedy Black Balls playing on the waiting room's TV was a welcome distraction. My mind drifted in and out of its comic banter. It was great to be laughing and smiling. All the same, I knew that soon the doors would be flung open and I would be escorted inside for an enema followed by the examination.

As usual the nurses were absolutely lovely, reassuring and kind. The enema worked efficiently—too efficiently perhaps as I felt the urge to go again when the anaesthetist drew back the curtain for his consultation. Even in those short few minutes I was once again struck by what a lovely guy he was. He had been my anaesthetist for the whopping 5.5 hour surgery! He even remembered I was a laughter facilitator and asked if I had returned to work.

My specialist, on the other hand, is solely focused on one part of me: my bowel. After numerous consultations both in his office and at my hospital bedside, I know he is far from impolite, in fact he is rather sweet and caring. Yet, sometimes, I wonder if all he sees when he looks at me is a jumbling of muscles and organs wrapped in skin, rather than the personality I've spent many years cultivating.

I have to remind myself that this seeming lack of interest in me is by no means a reflection of his capability as a surgeon, or his lack of care for me as a patient, as he has demonstrated more than clearly. I recall the skip in his stride and effusive smile from ear to ear when I asked if I could give him a kiss after he delivered the wonderful news we'd all been hoping to hear: that the cancer had not spread. There's no doubt whatsoever that I chose the best person for the job. Maybe pleasantries distract him from the important task at hand? I remind myself that I chose him for his finely attuned surgeon's hands earning him the affectionate nickname of 'Android'.

Still waiting to be admitted to the operating theatre, I began pondering the origin of the verb to heal which derives from the old English word hale meaning: to make whole, healthy or sound, to restore to health, free from ailment. In the company of my naturopath and other holistic practitioners a keen interest in my whole self is generally displayed. I feel validated and empowered, like healing is well within my capabilities. Yet in the presence of many other medical practitioners, aside from my father, brother and uncle, I often feel dissatisfied and frustrated at the lack of engagement in my personhood.

Philosophical meanderings ended as I was wheeled into the operating theatre. I glanced over at the surgeon, who was seated at the computer. He greeted my arrival in a courteous and polite manner. I didn't really register what he was saying, as in my head I was lost in imaginary dialogue. 'Ros, I've been expecting you,' delivered in an Austin Powers, as opposed to Godfather, voice. An IV was placed into my arm and my heart barely fluttered with this all-too-familiar procedure.

The next thing I knew I was waking up in the recovery room. The surgeon came by for what seemed like 10 seconds, but enough time to impart what he discovered. 'There's some inflammation around one of the titanium staples,' he said. 'It's very rare and I've never seen anything like it before, but it should resolve itself.' At least that's what my drugged and dazed head recalled. Then he was gone. That did seem like good news, although the 'should resolve itself' left me with a twinge of anxiety.

I psyched myself up to leave the recovery room when, beyond the curtain, another patient's voice relayed to a nurse they were waiting for a cab back to their flat in Woorigoleen St, Toorak. The street Booba (my grandmother) lived til her dying day. We were always amused by her pronunciation of 'Woorigoleen' in her thick Yiddish accent: 'Woollygoleen' or 'Worringollin'. I distinctly felt Booba's presence with me through this procedure and was grateful to have been alerted to this conversation. I mean what are the odds? Thank you for being with me Booba.

I went home a little worse for wear. I had missed school speech night. I really had missed it as Josh had been playing in the band although I was delighted to have had an excuse to miss the speech part. Sleep beckoned. After another long day, with the smell of hospital still lingering on my skin, I slipped under my sheets, which bore the distinctly sweet scent of home. Thank God I was home, safe and sound.

How important do you think it is for someone to demonstrate an interest in your whole self in terms of wellbeing?

....

....

....

If all your healing needs are not being met with one practitioner, consider supplementing your treatment plan with another practitioner, perhaps from a holistic background. We can't necessarily expect to get everything we need from just one person, but it is important to acknowledge what it is they do offer.

4 December 2011

Introductions please...

This evening, at a dinner party with very good friends, I was introduced to another guest in a manner that left me less than thrilled, 'And this is Ros. She's had more procedures in the past few months than anyone else I know.'

Great! What an introduction! Certainly one I could have done without and a claim to fame I would rather not own. I can't wait for the next time I'm back here or somewhere else and I'm introduced as, 'And this is Ros, my amazingly healthy and vibrant friend.' Now that kind of introduction I could get used to!

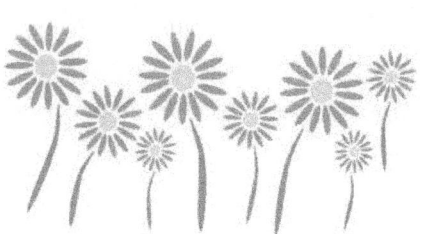

How would you like to be introduced in a new social setting?

....

....

....

10 December 2011
(Too) Great Expectations

I have come to the conclusion I have extremely high expectations in all (or most) aspects of my life. I expect my body to expeditiously heal and within the given time parameters. I expect shopping expeditions to be expertly and deftly carried out by Danny. I expect friends to rally around and enquire about my wellbeing. I expect to be given five minutes alone to write. So far this entry alone has already been interrupted twice. And by this, I don't even mean the intermittent licking of my feet by the house pooch … arghhh!

I expect to be offered a cup of tea if someone else is making one and for my plate to be cleared when another is being taken to the sink; for the neighbours to be considerate and not shout, scream or rev their quadruple exhausts at any given time of day or night.

I would like to say I expect, but it's more a desire (bordering on fantasy), for someone else to make dinner (and no, that does not include takeaways, although would that be such a bad thing?) Barely a night has gone by when dinner hasn't miraculously appeared on the table thanks to yours truly. As such I expect a small vote of thanks and appreciation, especially when it is evident magic does not just happen.

Is it wrong to have such high expectations? One thing for certain it does not make for merriment. I'm wondering whether expecting nothing and getting a little in return is better than expecting the world and getting scraps? Surely it is better to have higher expectations and lead by example?

I'm starting to think it's probably best to temper my expectations, not only of others, but also of myself. I need to be kinder on myself and give others an empathetic break. I need to relinquish some control. What I get, I get. What I give, I give. Importantly what I give and what I get are not as inextricably bound as a cause is to an effect. Focusing on people's inadequacies, as opposed to all the many and varied ways they are there for me, only leads to disappointment. Who knows, perhaps I am not living up to other people's expectations either?

I also need to apply this reasoning to my own healing. I will get better when I get better. Too high an expectation of the exact timing places too high a burden on my body to deliver something it simply is not ready for. It also diverts attention away from all the important healing that is already taking place.

I need to chill out, sit back and not work so hard at controlling and categorising everyone else according to how I view the world. This will lead to greater peace and serenity, less disappointment and an inner and outer world characterised by greater positivity, calm and delightful surprises.

'I will try not to expect so much from myself or from others.'

Do you have high expectations?

....

....

....

Do you have higher expectations of yourself or of others?

....

....

....

Discuss a time when your levels of expectations have not matched up to someone else's. How did that make you feel? How did you deal with it?

....

....

....

14 December 2011

A Love Story

Let love in.

Let love in are the words that keep coming to mind. I need to ingest, cogitate and meditate on these three words. Let love into my body even when I feel like cursing it. Let love into my life even when I'm drained. Especially when I'm drained.

Let love into every nook, every cranny, every cell, muscle and particle. Let it in, feel the love, let it rest until it permeates deeply. Let it dwell within, spilling out into daily chores, into the mundane, into every aspect of daily living. Let love in to enrich each living moment. Let love in to heal. Let love in to strengthen. Just let love in.

And now, as I'm considering what to write next, rather unexpectedly the Huey Lewis song from way back when, The Power of Love, starts blaring in my head, drowning out any substantive thoughts, so I may as well momentarily indulge my singing-self.

Anyway back on track. Love penetrates at a deep molecular level, through every living cell, drenching and quashing negativity, fear and sadness. If we could see love we would be blinded by its splendour. No one could dispute its power. Its expansiveness would speak for itself. And even though we can't touch it, it envelops us.

It's the penultimate bridge-builder connecting people, connecting worlds, and even linking universes. Just think about how you feel when you recall a loved one now departed. Love knows no boundaries or borders. It is goodness in the purest and most unadulterated form. It is a restorer of order stronger than any man–made physical manifestation. And while it is paramount to love other people, nothing is more important than the love we must hold for ourselves. If only we were trained at an early age to think in these terms and not feel sheepish or self-conscious uttering, 'I love you,' to ourselves. I am worthy of being loved. I am perfect just as I am. If only these words could take on a selfless guise, as I truly believe they were intended, devoid of self-centeredness and ego.

I welcome love. I invite love in. The gates of my heart are now truly open. I feel myself swelling in its richness. When I feel love, there is no other emotion; it's all empowering, all encompassing. I'm woozy in its spell as if I could float away inside its warm embrace to places far away.

I feel love. I am love. Without love, what is life?

My physical vibration has altered. I am calm. I am peace. I am basking in its magnificence. Love makes every cell in my body smile and glow. It is the medicine I need that cannot be prescribed. It is more powerful than any conventional or holistic practitioner. Basking in its glow makes me more youthful. Perhaps that explains the blissful look of meditators. How wondrous! How beneficent!

My heart is filled with love. My entire being is filled with love. I am love.

Affirmation time:
Every day, in every way I let love in
Every day, in every way I let love in
Every day, in every way I let love in.

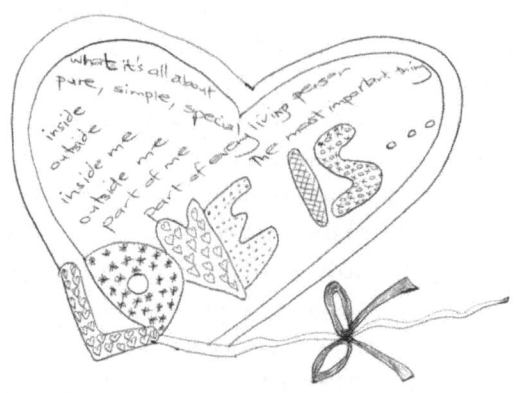

24 December 2011

Good butterflies in my stomach

I really can't believe it! Tomorrow we are leaving for Hong Kong and then on to Israel.

These words, 'Will she make it to Israel?' have popped into my head so many times these past seven or so months and have finally been answered. It's like a dramatic closing scene in an epic Hollywood movie, and I do love happy endings. I am so deeply grateful to be where I am right now. What a wonderful way to celebrate how much I have achieved this year physically, spiritually and emotionally.

Not only is this a big trip in its own right, it has served as a beacon of light at the end of a tunnel darkened by medical appointments, hospital stays, operations, uncertainties, anxieties and fear. A rocky road full of undulating twists and turns into the unknown. It is what I have ached for and dreamt about, holding numerous imaginary and real conversations. Celebrating Zak's Bar Mitzvah together with Danny's family in Israel is truly a dream come true; the ultimate reconnection with old friends and Israeli family, both distant and close. All treasured for the symbolism of what they represent: an interconnected past that we attempt to weave into our present. What a reward, not only for me, but also for my whole family, a real treat.

Not even in my darkest of moments did I relinquish this dream. The signs were always there, and if I wasn't looking hard enough, they'd appear even more boldly. Before the bowel reconnection we received an email from the travel agent enquiring if we still wanted him to hold our flights, leaving us mildly confused as we were certain we had cancelled them a few months before! Then the day before the reconnection came two other (non-spam) travel-related emails: one for discount travel insurance and the other offering a $500 travel voucher—both signs that gave me hope. I am so grateful my eyes have been open to these and other signs. They have illuminated what could have been a darkened path, beginning on the fateful day I received my permanent work contract and had my first CAT scan to investigate whether the cancer had spread.

Some signs were definitely more obvious than others. I'm actually giggling now as I remember stepping out our front door the day of my reconnection to go to the hospital to be immediately coated by a huge smattering of bird poo. Now in my upbringing being 'shat on' by birds is good luck, and since there had been an extra large dose, other than the inconvenience of having to change tops, I was quite delighted—definitely a good sign.

Now tomorrow has finally come. Suitcases expectantly line the corridor bulky with wintery clothes as we temporarily exit summer for the cooler, Northern Hemisphere winter. Yet inside I know I will be warm, spending time with family and friends. The mere thought of it warms the cockles of my heart, and has done so many times in the past, especially these last six months.

Thank you. Thank you. Thank you.

Israel, here we come!!

JOURNAL 4

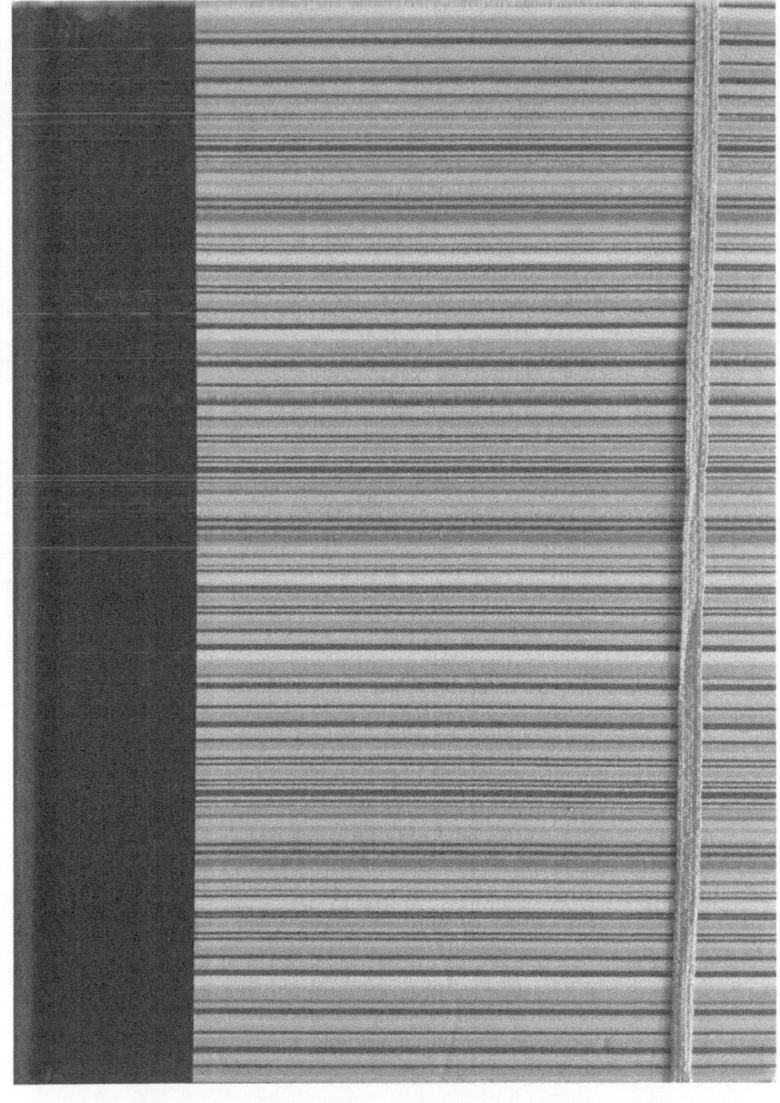

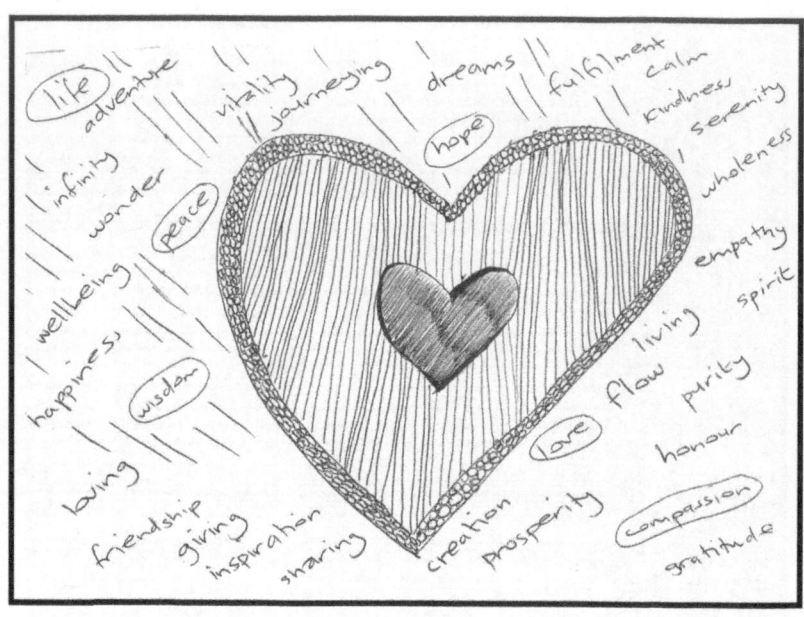

(Above: This love heart was inspired by a stunning ring worn by one of the shul-goers where Zak's Bar Mitzvah was held.)

31 December 2011
Jerusalem, Israel

Wow! We finally made it! This was the destination that provided me with much-needed hope, inspiration and an end goal. Lying in hospital beds, recuperating at home, in my sleep, dreams and meditation, this is where I dreamed and prayed we would all be, as a family, together in good health. Even though doubt clouded my vision many times during these long months somehow, deep inside I knew I'd make it. It just meant there was no room for complacency in my healing journey. I had to be well enough to travel.

My first taste of freedom was a three-night stopover in Hong Kong. Drunk on the gluttony of newfound experiences I tried tricking my physical body into being stronger than it was. I ignored my aching legs and heavy eyelids, filling them instead with new foods, experiences and sensations. It's not that I was foolhardy, I did slot some rest into my day, but in my enthusiasm I overdid things and the night before we were scheduled to fly to Israel I began feeling really unwell.

By morning I felt positively green. Our flight was at 4.30pm. I had to start feeling better. But no amount of positive talk could rouse my flailing energy levels. I could barely lift an arm or leg from my bed, let alone carry a suitcase on board or spend over 12 hours cramped in a pressurised economy cabin. What to do?

Once again, what I wanted to do and what I needed to do were diametrically opposed. I made the decision based on a hypothetical scenario of being offered a first class ticket on the afternoon flight. Nope, not even that could stir my depleted body. We would have to stay an extra night in Hong Kong and hopefully I would be well enough to travel the following evening.

Arrangements were made, credit cards whipp
charges for new flights and accommodation for a
a call-out Doctor provided me not only with a m
but one of the largest green pills I'd ever seen to

What else could be done? You can't fight gra
as I could not fight how I was feeling. Another
universe to slow down, take it easy, rest up.

'Hello Ros. Please listen to your inner voice.
Change your default position from yes to no, becaus
your body will leave you with no other choice tha
guilt-tripping yourself. Don't feel the desperate nee
anything all the time. FOMO (fear of missing out) i
will be a time for these things, but for now, no matter
wealth of experiences may be, your priority is to re
energy and allow the flow of vitality back into your b
blocks. Sit back. It will happen!'

Much love, t

Miraculously the next morning I felt mor
mustering enough energy to walk to the restau
graze on breakfast. I was conscious of each and e
moving in the right direction. I'm so grateful I
travel. We would all be able to travel.

I spent a quiet day soaking in the sun's warm
vibe of Hong Kong. In the evening we set off in
taxi with enough time ahead of the flight to secu
economy, all for myself! This flight was far empt
we were supposed to be on. The universe truly s
The 12+ hours passed easily enough. I even mana
or so hours in between stretching, wriggling and
to optimise blood flow. I am slightly paranoid ab
vein thrombosis (DVT) on planes having had on
years ago, but that's another story!

Finally the plane landed in the wee hours to a
of applause. Overcome with emotion, tears
Refraining from full-blown bawling was an effo

31 December 2011
Jerusalem, Israel

Wow! We finally made it! This was the destination that provided me with much-needed hope, inspiration and an end goal. Lying in hospital beds, recuperating at home, in my sleep, dreams and meditation, this is where I dreamed and prayed we would all be, as a family, together in good health. Even though doubt clouded my vision many times during these long months somehow, deep inside I knew I'd make it. It just meant there was no room for complacency in my healing journey. I had to be well enough to travel.

My first taste of freedom was a three-night stopover in Hong Kong. Drunk on the gluttony of newfound experiences I tried tricking my physical body into being stronger than it was. I ignored my aching legs and heavy eyelids, filling them instead with new foods, experiences and sensations. It's not that I was foolhardy, I did slot some rest into my day, but in my enthusiasm I overdid things and the night before we were scheduled to fly to Israel I began feeling really unwell.

By morning I felt positively green. Our flight was at 4.30pm. I had to start feeling better. But no amount of positive talk could rouse my flailing energy levels. I could barely lift an arm or leg from my bed, let alone carry a suitcase on board or spend over 12 hours cramped in a pressurised economy cabin. What to do?

Once again, what I wanted to do and what I needed to do were diametrically opposed. I made the decision based on a hypothetical scenario of being offered a first class ticket on the afternoon flight. Nope, not even that could stir my depleted body. We would have to stay an extra night in Hong Kong and hopefully I would be well enough to travel the following evening.

Arrangements were made, credit cards whipped out to cover charges for new flights and accommodation for an extra night, and a call-out Doctor provided me not only with a medical certificate, but one of the largest green pills I'd ever seen to assist digestion.

What else could be done? You can't fight gravity, just as much as I could not fight how I was feeling. Another lesson from the universe to slow down, take it easy, rest up.

'Hello Ros. Please listen to your inner voice. Learn to say no. Change your default position from yes to no, because in the long run your body will leave you with no other choice than to say no. No guilt-tripping yourself. Don't feel the desperate need to be a part of anything all the time. FOMO (fear of missing out) is overrated! There will be a time for these things, but for now, no matter how tempting the wealth of experiences may be, your priority is to rest, replenish your energy and allow the flow of vitality back into your body. Don't put up blocks. Sit back. It will happen!'

Much love, the Universe xxx

Miraculously the next morning I felt more human, even mustering enough energy to walk to the restaurant and lightly graze on breakfast. I was conscious of each and every step but was moving in the right direction. I'm so grateful I would be able to travel. We would all be able to travel.

I spent a quiet day soaking in the sun's warm rays and bustling vibe of Hong Kong. In the evening we set off in a luggage-laden taxi with enough time ahead of the flight to secure three seats in economy, all for myself! This flight was far emptier than the one we were supposed to be on. The universe truly smiled upon me. The 12+ hours passed easily enough. I even managed to sleep five or so hours in between stretching, wriggling and moving around to optimise blood flow. I am slightly paranoid about getting deep vein thrombosis (DVT) on planes having had one in my leg four years ago, but that's another story!

Finally the plane landed in the wee hours to a subdued round of applause. Overcome with emotion, tears filled my eyes. Refraining from full-blown bawling was an effort. I had arrived in the place of my dreams and the collective dreams and prayers of so many. I was so extraordinarily grateful. What an achievement. What a journey! I had done so well!

Do you hear and respond to your inner voice?

....

....

....

If you haven't listened, have there been any consequences? If so, what were they?

....

....

....

Is there a message your inner voice is telling you now?

....

....

....

3 January 2012

Heaven on Earth

Today was the most amazing day, really perfect. The closer we got to the Kotel (Western Wall) in Jerusalem, the more sounds permeated the crisp winter air: the beat of drums, the hypnotic chanting of prayer—amidst the general hubbub of activity. A common day for Bar Mitzvahs, outside of the Sabbath, the forecourt of the Kotel could have been mistaken for a colourful chessboard, from a distance—a mosaic of head coverings and robes. Huddles of smartly dressed boys from all corners of the world congregated here: gold-bedecked boys of Yemenite background, others with black hats ensconced in a sea of taller hats and secular Israeli boys wearing signature T-shirts and jeans. The air was filled with such joy and celebration that a Richter scale could have imploded from all the seen and felt emotion.

Making my way to the women's section of the Kotel, I squeezed in between a multitude of arms, hands and heads and pressed my forehead and two palms to this ancient wall. I recited the Shema (one of the most symbolic and powerful of prayers, 'Hear, O Israel, the Lord our God, the Lord is One') and before I could determine what to do next, my eyes welled with tears. Contemplating the year that had been I wanted to pray for an easier and healthier future. The word that immediately came to me was brachot (blessings). I wanted lots of brachot, for them to rain down upon my loved ones and myself, to be drenched and saturated by them.

As I uttered my deepest and innermost prayer for blessings, tears from the very core of my being and essence surfaced. First trickling, then streaming. There was nothing forced in these tears.

I did not even feel uncomfortable or self-conscious in releasing such depths of emotion in the company of strangers. My own tears blended with those of the countless others who had been here before me over the course of centuries. I was deeply connected to a sense of timeless yearning and healing.

Being here was what I had dreamed about, when I had lied petrified, wrapped in silver waist-down in the pre-operating cubicle, awaiting the first operation. It was here I was transported when my surgeon delivered the great news that deep down I already knew: the cancer had not spread and I would be fine.

I was lost in emotion. Should I be asking for anything else? What if I drowned in my tears? Perhaps I could have stayed a little longer, prayed a little harder, but with both sleeves I wiped away my streaming tears. Tears that had been gestating for so long; tears filled with fear, grief and all things unknown. They had now been released from my physical and spiritual body. I could now move on. And that's exactly what I did, both metaphorically and literally. Still facing the wall, slowly and deliberately I walked backwards.

I left this holy dumping ground, a place of unmet and met prayers and miracles, and re-entered a space of celebration, of Mazel Tovs, ululating Yemenite women, drums beating together with chanting and clapping, signalling the momentous leap from boyhood to manhood. The next generation still bathed in innocence and wrapped in youth.

Before this day I had never really felt the awesomeness (in the literal sense) of the Kotel. I had known what I was supposed to feel, but it had taken a brush with the fragility of human life to discover a new aspect of my emotional self. Now my connection to this self was stronger. This was the connection I needed to listen to, to nurture and to obey. It would keep me safe and strong and ultimately guide me on my path of Truth. Dare I veer again.

I am now intimately connected to my feeling self, and with it to my emotions. I must not suppress this aspect of myself. I must learn to express it, to listen and be guided by it. I need to ensure other people's truths do not cloud or suppress mine or influence me into bearing a weight that is theirs. I need to turn off external voices pressuring me into feeling or not feeling something in a particular way, akin to trampling on a living thing. Of course we are all shaped by multiple influences, but danger resides when these voices become louder than our own.

On previous visits to the Kotel, I had been filled with other people's notions of how I should feel, based on how they felt, or supposed one should feel in a place of awe. But forcing a feeling amounts to not feeling at all. I had borrowed so many of my feelings from others, denying myself the opportunity to explore how I could and should express my own truth. Over a lifetime I had become detached from my inner feelings. I reined them in, in the name of control, sensibility and perceived societal expectations. Yet now I owned my feelings. I had transformed into a feeling being.

Through the tears shed by my feeling self, rawness was finally exposed. What a release! What a relief! I became aware of the deep, symbolic meaning the Kotel held for so many people over such a long time-span. I don't know which symbol or place holds similar meaning for people of other faiths and it does not matter, as long as it's there. A place to direct your prayers, to journey to (both in your mind and physically), a place that holds spiritual fortitude. Your own special place. And with that I say Amen.

What special place do you have?

....

....

....

If one does not come to mind, spend some time meditating on one now. Look deep within. Remember it's your special place.

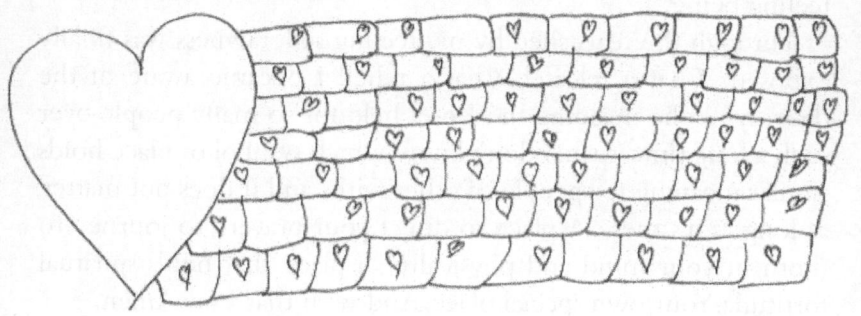

(Above: Kotel [Wall] of Love)

23 January 2012
Zak's Bar Mitzvah

The day I had been waiting for finally arrived. Hearing Zak recite his Bar Mitzvah portion, his sweet voice permeating the stone walls of Jerusalem's oldest synagogue, was incredibly surreal. In the past year, these ancient words have echoed around our house, at times filtering from the upstairs living room during dedicated lessons, occasionally being heard garbled by the shower's steady trickle and even silently rehearsed by Zak's lips as they streamed from his iPhone. But never could I have imagined this. Several times during the service, I caught myself peaking at the old city shimmering in the distance, momentarily becoming lost in its timeless beauty. I kept urging myself to be present, to be truly present. I don't understand why I thought I was not. Most likely it was the enormity of the occassion. I hoped bringing a level of awareness would precipitate my conscious state into being fully present. This was most definitely a moment I wanted to savour. It had certainly been a helluva long road getting here, and not just from Melbourne to Jerusalem!

It's interesting that even whilst writing this entry I am still not fully clear about what it means to be truly present. How many moments pass each day without acknowledgment, disappearing without a trace as though they had never come to be? It's hard defining being present, but to me it can also be quite simple:

Being aware and focused, taking in and appreciating the present moment with all senses heightened. Being present is when time stops or slows down even if only for a few conscious seconds, when one transitions from a state of doing to being.

So many times in the past six months this has been more dream than reality. Where flights have been booked, cancelled and 'rebooked'. As for the synagogue booking, we held off paying the deposit for as long as possible, whilst Danny and the extraordinarily patient administrator and Rabbi corresponded with progress updates. Last week when we met them for the first time face-to-face it was like connecting with old friends. They were more aware of what had been going on these past few months in our personal life than many of our known compatriots.

Staring around at this congregation was quite surreal. It was so familiar yet so foreign, so filled with love. We were accompanied by my inherited family from the UK: mother-in-law, father-in-law, sister-in-law, brother-in-law, Danny's aunt, uncle and cousin as well as relatives' friends from Israel and Australian friends who just happened to be in Israel. As much as I dearly wished my parents, siblings, and closest friends could have joined us, it just hadn't been possible. We couldn't expect others to commit to a trip we weren't even sure we would ourselves make. We had confirmed only a few weeks in advance—a record even for us.

In any case, it was perfect just the way it was. The temperature outside may have been close to zero, but I was submerged in warmth emanating from the depths of my soul. Zak delivered his part to perfection and was showered with not only love but as tradition dictates, lots of sweets.

After the service, around forty guests shared a festive lunch. The room was filled with friends and family, and my heart with love and wonder. One of the invitees, an older distant family friend, came over and asked if I knew how the family was connected. Other than recalling his family shared a friendship with my late grandparents in Germany, I didn't know any specifics and was silently hoping he wasn't expecting me to fill a gap in his knowledge. He then excitedly told me his father was a doctor on the battlefields of WW1 Germany, where my grandfather delivered food to battle-fatigued soldiers on the frontline. My grandfather had been shot and it was this man's father who saved his life, extracting the bullet and delivering him to safety.

I was absolutely gobsmacked. Had it not been for his father's heroic acts, my grandfather might not have gone on to be the man he became, marry, bear my mother and I wouldn't be here. My grandfather was awarded the Iron Cross for his bravery, and I hoped this man's heroics had also been rewarded. What a debt of gratitude we owe to this family! Incredible!

These memories will live inside me forever. I am so very grateful to everyone who has helped make this a giant of a day. To the three men in my family: Danny, Josh and now Zak, thank you for giving meaning and purpose to my life beyond any wild imaginings. I am so proud of you all in different ways, but mostly because you fill not only my heart, but also the hearts of so many others with joy, love and laughter. May you continue to shine your very own special light now and forever.

xoxo

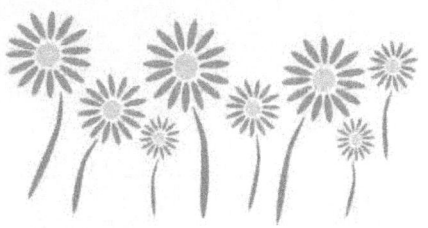

What does being present mean to you?

....

....

....

Recount a time you felt truly present.

....

....

....

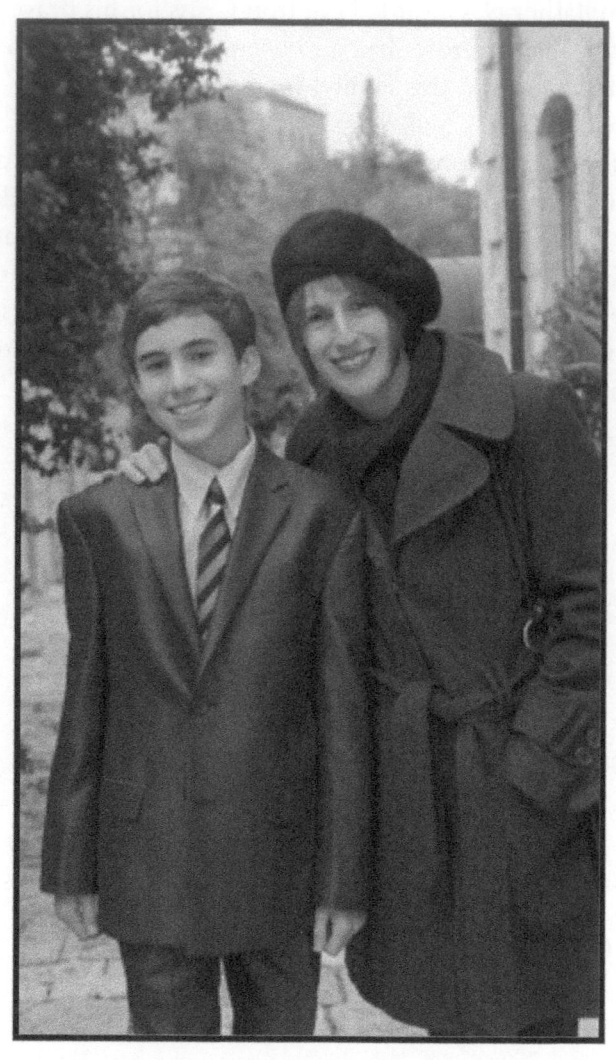

(Above: Ros and Zak outside Beit Yisrael Synagogue, Yemin Moshe, Jerusalem)

9 March 2012

Am I a cancer 'survivor'?

I'm almost beginning to question if there's something in the air or water. Ever since my return from Israel so many friends have been diagnosed with some sort of cancer: ovarian, breast, skin, just to name a few. It's actually got to the point that if a friend calls, especially if I haven't spoken to them in a while, I momentarily hold my breath in dread until I hear the words, 'All is well.'

Just now I have been engaged in a series of text communiqués with an acquaintance who I recently learned has aggressive breast cancer. Contained in her latest message were the words, 'I am now a member of the cancer survivor club, like you.'

Hold on a second ... I'm not a cancer survivor. I just had a cancerous polyp removed, which happened to entail some rather major surgeries. I thank God I didn't have to go through chemotherapy or radiation. Nup, I'm no survivor.

But these words won't leave my mind. Could I or should I be classified as a survivor of cancer? What are the criteria? How much suffering and how many interventions do you need to undergo to be classified as one? How would someone who has nearly lost his or her life to cancer, or undergone far more radical treatment than myself, view my being a survivor? Couldn't it be regarded as a bit of an insult to what they have gone through as 'real survivors'?

I am grappling with the use of war metaphors around cancer: survivors; she lost the battle; he's a real battler; she's a real hero; she was so brave; he lost his brave fight. Even pharmaceutical companies and cancer researchers have joined the bandwagon with such phrases as waging the war against cancer. The problem with this terminology is the underlying inference of guilt or failure if someone with cancer can't defeat this affliction; even though I'm sure that's the last thing anyone would consciously want to convey.

To an extent, bravery implies a choice and who really has a choice in getting or not getting cancer? I imagine most people who endure cancer treatment regimens (even I am succumbing to the war terminology) would not view themselves as heroes; they're just doing whatever they need to optimise their chance of healing and survival, indubitably in flag bearing mode.

For some, the idea of a fight or a battle is motivating, but for others it could be equally damaging. I'm struggling to think of other diseases or afflictions that draw on war terminology. The only other context I'm used to hearing survivor terminology is for holocaust survivors. I wonder whether here too there is some ambiguity around this issue. For some, a person who's been through a concentration camp may be viewed as a true survivor, but perhaps another person who faced significant hardship, but not as extreme, may not? To my knowledge, anyone who endured these years of terror and came out alive is referred to as a holocaust survivor. Maybe amongst this demographic too, judgment around who qualifies as a 'real survivor' exists, just like I'm positing with regards to cancer.

As for me, in deference to other people I consider to be true cancer survivors, undergoing chemo and the works, I'm disassociating myself from the survivor label. It really makes me feel uncomfortable. Also I don't want to maintain an association to this particular episode any longer than I need to, and referring to myself as a survivor maintains some level of attachment. This is one club membership I'm not hankering for. I want to be defined by all the positive things I create in my life, and not that one incy wincy polyp that caused a great deal of pain, trauma and havoc.

What criteria do you think are needed to classify as a survivor?

....
....
....

If you have had a particular illness (cancer or something else) do you
refer to yourself as a survivor?

....
....
....

How does that term make you feel?

....
....
....

30 May 2012
My 44th Birthday

A wonderful birthday celebration compensating for the last one spent in the surgeon's office.

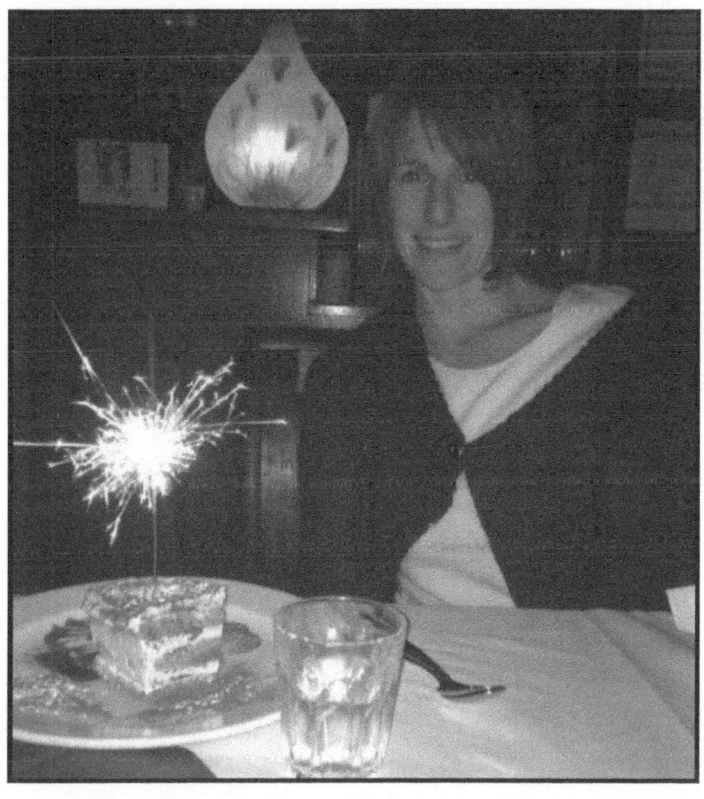

15 June 2012

Do only nice people get cancer?

I'm two days short of my one-year anniversary since the bowel resection and truly marvel at time's passing. I'm feeling exceedingly lucky, but especially in the context of so many new cancer diagnoses around me and the recent, very sad death of a friend from tertiary breast cancer.

But what really irks me is what appears to be the standard response to a new cancer diagnosis. It often involves something like this: 'Did you hear so and so has cancer. They're so nice ... always helping others. It just doesn't seem fair.'

I want to know: SINCE WHEN DOES BEING NICE PRECLUDE YOU FROM CANCER? I hope you heard me shouting! Anyway it got me thinking. Could it be possible that only nice people get cancer? So I went to the most logical place to get answers: Google. Initially I was befuddled by the horoscope information topping the list of searches, but then it dawned on me, cancer is not just a disease; it's also a star sign! How funny!

It turns out there have been extensive studies on personality traits as risk and prognostic factors for cancer. I'd certainly heard about Type A personality but Type C personality was news to me. And the bizarre thing is until I read further I assumed that the C stood for cancer, which it doesn't. The C is allocated as the alphabetical letter next in line after the two better-known personality types: A and B.

Type C is indicative of someone at heightened risk for assorted health issues ranging from colds and other viral or bacterial infections to cancer. They contrast sharply to Type A people who are often believed to be prime candidates for cardiovascular disease owing to their competitive, achievement-oriented, often impatient personality. Then there's Type B people who are much more relaxed and reflective. I think I have B-Type envy.

One of the leaders in this field of research, Lydia Temoshok, PhD,[6] describes a Type C person as a pleaser who spends much of his or her existence trying to be accepted by others. Her research began in 1979 on patients with melanoma along with many commonly observed personality traits. The first group she identified consisted of patients who were more worried about the effect a cancer diagnosis was having on their families than on themselves.

I'm beginning to feel a little uneasy as that was exactly how I first reacted, and where, to an extent, I still concern myself. And it gets worse. Three quarters of research participants (and this study has since been replicated by other researchers) exhibited the following behaviours: repressed emotions, not displaying anger, past or present. They tended to not experience or express any other negative emotions such as fear, anxiety or sadness. They were patient, unassertive, disliked conflict, overly concerned with meeting other people's needs, and often prone to self-sacrificing to an extreme.

Tick, tick, tick, tick and tick. Oh f**k. I'm screwed!

I kept reading as though I was watching an unexpectedly violent film with my eyes half-covered but unable to fully turn away. Thankfully there was some good news. Patients who were more emotionally expressive had thinner tumours, more slowly dividing cancerous cells and a higher number of lymphocytes (immune cells) invading the tumour. Conversely patients who were less emotionally expressive had thicker tumours and more rapidly dividing cancer cells, with significantly fewer lymphocytes invading the tumour.

Clearly intuiting how others like I, a freshly out-of-the-closet C-Type, would feel reading this research, the author had written the following in a big, bold font: 'Avoiding self-blame and guilt'.

---

6   Temoshok, L., Unraveling the 'Type C' Connection: Is There a Cancer Personality? Implications for Prevention & Recovery (http://www.healingcancer.info/ebook/lydia-temoshok)

She explained:

'No-one can be blamed for mind-body factors in cancer, because no one intentionally develops the cancer-prone behaviour pattern. Furthermore without knowledge of the Type C cancer link how could someone realise that his/her behaviour might impact his cancer defence system on a molecular level?'

My brain could barely keep up as my eyes darted ahead. I was hooked; totally riveted by the prospect of further revelations. I was right, as nestled in between more statistics, Temoshok stated the following.

'Type C behaviour had been each person's best attempt to cope with the pains, stresses, humiliations and unmet needs of early childhood.'

But in order to realise later in life that these no longer served an individual well, first, one needed to become aware of this, only then could one make any necessary adjustments.

So there is hope. I can change. I can be less nice, or in other words prioritise my own self-care. I can express a differing opinion in a way that doesn't exacerbate conflict—just a difference of opinion. I can express my anger in a healthful way. Perhaps I can even laugh my anger and frustrations away? I don't have to be so preoccupied with my perception of how others see me. At the end of the day it's what I think of myself that counts. I need to be brave enough to believe that this is more than enough. I'm always the first person to stand up if I witness any unfairness or injustice; I need to apply the same rules to myself.

I keep searching for more information about the C-Type. Another researcher, the Canadian physician Gabor Maté[7], offers an explanation on the link between being nice and being more prone to getting cancer. Here's what he says.

'When an individual engages in a long-term practice of ignoring or suppressing legitimate feelings, i.e. when he or she is just plain too nice, the immune system can become compromised and confused, learning to attack the self rather than defend it.' 3

7   Maté, G. (2003). When the Body Says No – Exploring the Stress Disease Connection, John Wiley & sons, New Jersey.

According to Maté, emotional expression is absolutely essential. 'Feelings serve to alert the individual to what is dangerous or unwholesome – or, conversely, to what is helpful and nourishing – so that the person can either take protective action against the thread or move toward the beneficial stimulus. If someone never gets angry, this reflects an unhealthy inability or unwillingness to defend personal integrity'.

If someone just cannot say no, he concludes, his or her body will end up expressing it in the form of illness or disease. Incredible! That's me too! I hate saying no to people. I'm a classic 'I'll do it' person, and love helping out until my plate overflows as I topple under its weight. It's more a matter of calling than choice.

I once adopted an elderly gentleman whose wife had passed on and his only daughter lived on the other side of the world. Over the course of many years my nuclear family became his family. I got a grandfather, and my kids, a great-grandfather. Sadly he has since passed on. Then there was a former neighbour with chronic schizophrenia and a host of other issues to whom, outside of family members, I became the sole connection. I loved becoming a part of these two souls' lives and the mostly seamless process of joining another family, of being there for them, but as much as these experiences were phenomenally enriching, they also depleted my precious energy reserves.

As my family will testify, my helping streak occasionally verges on extreme. Just now in Israel as I was approaching some pedestrian lights I spotted an elderly lady in the distance slowly pushing her shopping trolley up the gentle slope. My eyes almost glazed over, as I thought how much I missed not helping anyone, especially someone elderly. Then out of the blue her trolley tumbled, along with her groceries, and yours truly escorted her (bags and all) back to her apartment. Apologies to this lovely lady if somehow my helping vibes got a little out of control!

The problem with my inability to say no is that I overdo it and then am no use to anyone. My mother-in-law Lillian is always reminding me, 'You are made of the cloth you're given and no matter how much you want to do something, if that's all you've got to work with, then that's all you've got.'

I'm going to have to take on board everything I've just read. Naturally, there's far more to getting cancer than being a particular personality type, but it has given me food for thought. I have to learn to say no, to take care of myself, as no one else can do it on my behalf. I have to explore other, more healthful ways to help people and be the kind of person I want to be. I'm so grateful to have this knowledge as I can now conscientiously create new behavioural patterns to enhance and support my wellbeing.

Definitely time for some affirmations:

My needs are just as important as anyone else's
I can and must express ALL my emotions, not just the positive ones
I don't always have to be preoccupied with other people's needs
I don't have to avoid conflict at all cost
I don't need to conform if I feel strongly about something
I don't need to be a martyr!
I need to cherish and promote my own value and worth.

What personality type are you?

....
....
....

Are there certain attributes about your personality that you recognise to be unhealthful or damaging to your wellbeing? If so, what are they and in what way/s can you change?

....
....
....

19 June 2012

One year CT Scan

'I'll be fine; you really don't need to come with me. It's just a scan, you don't have to miss your meeting,' was what I told Danny last night before today's CT scan.

Famous last words, as I nervously traipsed the nuclear medicine corridors, aching for a hand to hold. An assembly of whirring machines fuelled by nuclear power, alien catacombs. As the gown slipped over my head I metamorphosed into a patient. I couldn't stop shaking which posed a minor challenge for the nurse trying to fit an IV bung into my vein. Well in theory I had veins—they had to be hiding somewhere.

I have grown used to the fortnightly rectal examinations, but being asked to submit to the jaws of the CT scanner thrust me straight into fear. Moments became ultra-spaced out as two technicians struggled to find a suitable vein to feed the radioactive dye. Finally success was marked by the disquieting feeling of having wet myself, as I was propelled in, and then out of the tunnel. A robotic voice boomed, 'Breathe in, then hold. Breathe in, then hold'. I was fake-breathing, hoping to get away with it, as to really breathe in this space was impossible. Thankfully the desired outcome was attained and I was free to go. I did not need a mirror to relay a complexion as pale as the gown, but no one remarked on it.

Clothes back on, IV bung out and with a pounding heart I raced towards the hospital exit sign as quickly as I could without breaking into a run. I just wanted to run. To be immersed in normalcy. I was craving to be held and thought perhaps if I headed to my local supermarket I might bump into a friend as so often did happen. I didn't, but just knowing I was free to go where I wanted to and do what I wanted helped me return to a more even keel. That, and I decided to treat myself and detoured past one of my favourite bakeries for a cake I could savour with a nice cup of tea in the comfort of my own home.

One thing I can say with certainty is that was anything other than 'just a scan'. Now the next thing to tick off my 12-month review is next week's colonoscopy.

If you have had a rough day, why not squeeze in a little treat for yourself? What sort of things might you do?

....

....

....

2 July 2012
Sitting small opposite the big man

'I'll be fine; you really don't need to come with me. It's just a follow up appointment, you don't have to miss any work,' was what I told Danny before my appointment with the surgeon. I am wondering if I'm having déjà-vu as I'm sure these were nearly the exact same words I uttered just over a week ago before my CT scan. Yep, I just checked my last entry and they were. I definitely have an over-developed independent streak!

Danny delivering and collecting me for the colonoscopy had been a non-issue. The nursing staff treated me with kid gloves not knowing that for me a colonoscopy was an absolute doddle after what I had been through. Lying in the recovery room the surgeon informed me that everything looked great, so what else could I hope for? Today was just a routine follow-up appointment. I really didn't need my hand held. Once again, famous last words.

'Your scan looks good other than something showing on your liver. I don't recall anything being there last year when we did the scan,' the surgeon started. 'Probably nothing to worry about. Just a liver cyst. Is your referral to the gastroenterologist still valid?' he asked but continued before I could answer. 'I recommend you make an appointment so he can take a closer look and advise further steps if necessary. But other than that, it all looks good. The bowel and assorted seams have healed well. Any concerns?' he asked. With a slightly sunken heart, I numbly shook my head. 'OK good, see you in a fortnight.'

Once again I felt two inches tall. Well maybe two feet. Then in a dazed state I transported myself to my car and drove home. To be honest I can't even remember driving home but safe to say I must have. The first thing I did was something I never should have done—typed liver cyst into Google which immediately delivered a listing of everything liver + cyst: liver cysts and tumours, benign tumours and cystic disease, and so the list went on. Of course, what I didn't want to see was any mention of cancer, but I soon discovered that even though most cysts are benign, in some instances they are or become malignant. As I didn't even know if that was what I had, my search grew a little farther until I shouted out aloud 'STOP!' putting a moratorium on any further investigations. Then with a trembling hand I reached out for the phone to call my gastroenterologist. As luck would have it a 3pm appointment two days later had just become available.

Fast forward to my appointment with the gastroenterologist, once again on my lonesome for some really good reason I've already forgotten. He played down what in my mind had already escalated to a full-blown medical emergency, explaining that liver cysts were in the majority of cases benign and jokingly adding that they were so common they were one of the main reasons he was in business. Taking a closer look at my scan he seemed relatively confident that's what it was, but an MRI would be able to show more conclusively. Given the amounts of radiation I had recently been exposed to, he recommended I get it done some time in the next three months. He shot me a look of sympathy and said, 'Try and not concern yourself too much about it.'

As reassuring and well-intended as these sentiments may have been, they did little to quell my anxiety, but I promised I would try and put it to the back of my mind and not think about it, at least for a couple of months.

So that's what I'm trying to do this very moment. Not think about it. My lips start to quiver and my eyes fill with tears as I imagine Danny walking in the door, but until then, with the kids in earshot, I will stay strong. I need to distract myself and a hovering pooch provides the perfect solution. I'm going out for some fresh air and a walk.

List 3 things that went well in your day

Years ago I attended a happiness workshop with founder of Positive Psychology, Dr Martin Seligman, author of Authentic Happiness.[5] His research, which has since been substantiated, found the 'Three Good Things' (also known as 'Three Blessings') exercise to be an effective strategy to enhance individual happiness and wellbeing.

So, as I lie on the cusp of sleep, I recall or compile a list of three things that went well in my day. You can either compose this list in your head or write it down in a notebook. If you choose to write it down, when you're feeling down you can easily refer back to all these things. You will be amazed at how much you have to be grateful for!

Things that went well in your day can range from a great catch up with a friend, to a good test result or even some uninterrupted time spent outside with the sun on your skin. It's about focusing on some of the small things that happened in your day that made you feel good, not just the big things such as a work promotion. It's very difficult to remain in a negative state of mind when you are focusing on something positive. In fact it can be quite addictive; you might not be able to stop at three! That's why I love doing this practice in the evening because it optimises my chances of falling into a peaceful slumber and with a smile on my face.

---

5   Seligman, M.E.P., Authentic Happiness: Using the New Positive Psychology to Realize Your Potential for Lasting Fulfillment. New York: Free Press. 2004

5 September 2012
Mid-Semester Blues

After a particularly long day, I came home in the late afternoon, eager to chill out and watch something relatively inane on TV, but I had been beaten to the couch, and the news was blaring into our living room. Rather than demand the channel be changed, I extricated myself from accounts of death and destruction to the confines of my room and this journal. I'm quite proud of myself!

Now to the subject of work … I'm like a hologram, a hollow projection. Physically I'm in the lecture theatre, but my heart and soul are not. I go through the motions of sounding passionate about the teachings I am imparting, but my passion for the subject matter has been decommissioned. It's not that the teachings are not interesting, relevant or important, because they most definitely are. It's just not my talk; it's someone else's. My truth, my heart now resides in all things healing, laughter and wellness.

I am also acutely aware of my energy reserves and what replenishes or drains them. At the end of the teaching day, I am exhausted, driving home marred with blurred vision. Yet, on days I facilitate mindfulness or laughter sessions I'm perfectly at peace or soaring on a happy high.

I recall how I stumbled into this academic life, when three years ago a conversation about the possibility of some sessional work led to a sudden leap into the abyss. The Health Promotion subject coordinator had abruptly resigned and the department was in dire need to fill the position (the words that come to mind are 'up shit creek without a paddle') with a new semester beginning in just two weeks. In between jobs and with slight trepidation I agreed to step in. Things progressed well, resulting in my being offered a permanent position last May, during that fateful week, providing me with the best sign I could possibly have hoped for: a future!

Yet now I am distracted, constructing lists of pros and cons: go it alone with my company LaughLife or remain teaching at university? Quite frankly university is not coming out on top. I still absolutely love the interaction with students. I mean that's why I am there. And then there's the financial reliability and even the potential to develop my own course Laughter, Wellbeing and Happiness dangling like a carrot in front of my face. But then there's the hour-long commute, huge assessment load, bureaucratic hoops and increasing reliance on visual technology to replace human interaction. My wings have been clipped and I ache to soar.

With the liver cyst fresh in my mind, and the slow unravelling of the year that was, I'm struggling with the university load emotionally and physically. Although I take solace knowing that the end of the year is nigh.

When was the last time you had a news-free day?

....

....

....

News is rarely uplifting, so perhaps consider burying your head in the sand for a while. Or even better, construct your own list of good news items to share with others.

....

....

....

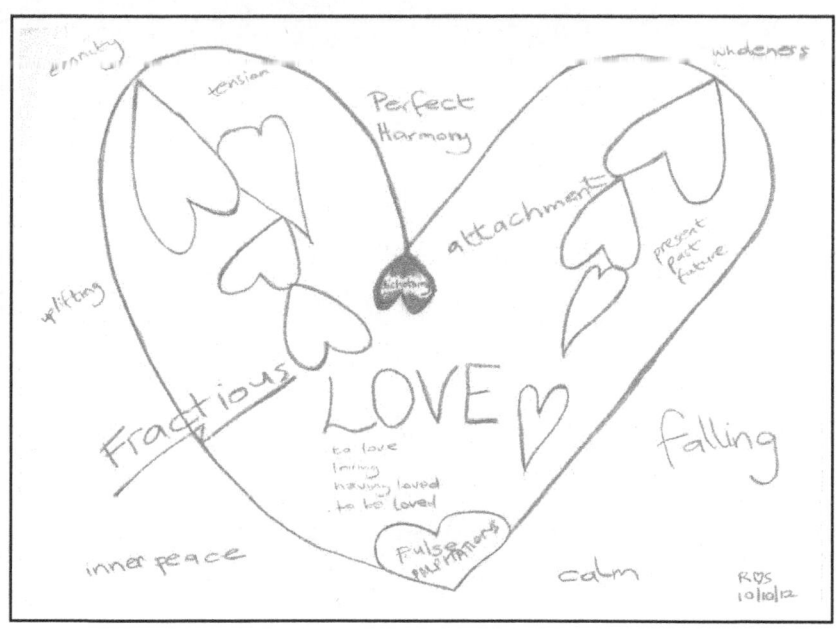

'Love' 14 October 2012

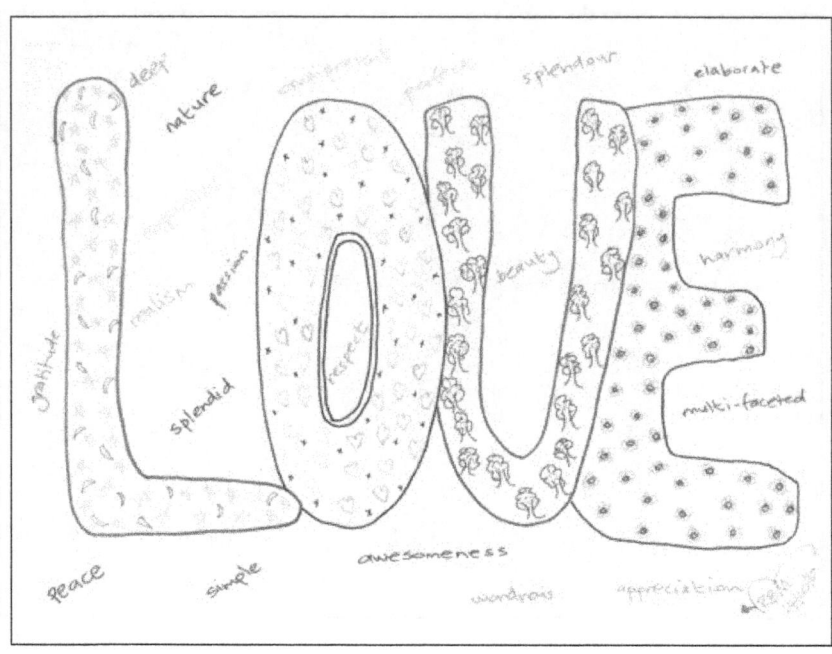

14 October 2011
Just Breathe...

Each morning before the first light, my racing heart stirs me. The silence is deafening, disrupted only by my thumping heart. No matter how relaxed I am when I retire, during the course of the evening I wake prematurely as if I have run a marathon, minus the health benefits.

I lie, then toss and turn with mounting frustration. I envy Danny's deep sleep, his occasional snore or even snortle. I wonder which dream domain he inhabits. Quiet as a mouse I suck in slow and deep breaths cautious not to disturb him. I will myself back to sleep, back to my own dream domain, but that in itself is not enough. Sleep still eludes and soon my frustration verges on anger.

In these cruel hours I try tricking my frazzled state into one of calm. I'm at the beach, on a mountain or gazing into a calm sapphire lake. Yet no matter how serene the image, my inner self won't fall for them. The newly discovered liver cyst has stopped my breathing right in its tracks. Shadowing the anxious tempo of my pulsating heart, it is momentarily stuck between my diaphragm and mouth.

This is how it has been for the past week or so and I'm absolutely exhausted, fed up and am bad company all around. My patient streak has been halted. I can't stop snapping at everyone. I think about people who wish they could sleep like a baby. People instead should wish they breathed like a baby—the perfect breathing vessel—belly rising and falling, deeply and slowly, naturally and peacefully. My current breathing pattern is all over the place.

At present all I want to do is stay close to my couch to rest, breathe and meditate. This isn't indulgence; it's survival. I'm addicted to mindful breathing. It's all I want to do. In these moments of slowing and deepening my breaths I derive such benefit, sometimes ephemeral, other times longer. Breathing deeply frees my parasympathetic nervous system from being hijacked by its oppressor, the sympathetic nervous system. It empowers it. Yet try as I might, peace is nowhere to be found, least of all within me.

I need to do something to break this cycle. I decide to up the ante and become a daytime mindful breathing devotee. I have to or I will be engulfed. I appreciate now that the way we breathe fulfils so much more than a functional life-preserving role. By equal measure it can calm or it can storm. Without it we are nothing.

Deep breathing is one of the fastest and most effective ways to bring peace and calm to my two warring nervous systems and find balance. That expiration (big sigh) moment as peace is welcomed in by my parasympathetic and stress is escorted away from my sympathetic nervous system. It will just take dedicated time and practice.

At least I have cultivated some level of awareness. I just caught myself holding my breath writing this. So, time now to sign off and take a long breather.

How do you usually breathe?

Whilst standing, place one hand on your chest and one on your belly. Take a deep breath in and then out (through your nose or mouth) and observe which hand moves more. Does your breath stem more from your chest or your belly?

Practice breathing with your diaphragm, which is a bit like a balloon and sits between your lower rib cage and abdomen, so the hand on your belly moves more. It can feel a bit counter-intuitive as when you breathe deeply in your belly pops out and when you breathe out it pops back in.

Breathing exercises I found helpful during times of anxiety

Choose any of these breathing exercises and practice once or twice a day for at least 15 minutes. It is really important to find a method that works best for you. You can even alternate practices depending on mood and setting. Setting a timer is beneficial as then you don't have to disrupt your practice to look at the time.

Rhythmic Breathing
Great for balancing your parasympathetic and sympathetic nervous systems, in rhythmic breathing you inhale for the same count as you exhale (out the nose or mouth).

Begin by sitting upright in a comfortable position. Close your eyes and place your hands on your belly. You want to encourage breathing from your abdomen, because when you're more stressed your breath tends to stem from the chest. Breathing from your abdomen activates the parasympathetic nervous system and a relaxation response.

Breathe in for a count of 5, and then exhale for a count of 5. If you can, inhale and exhale for a longer count comfortable for you. Pause (for as long as it takes to say 'pause') after each breath cycle (in and out) to maintain control of your breath. With practice you will find you can breathe in and out for a longer count. Once you have engaged abdominal breathing you can rest your hands by your side. Continue this process for 15 minutes and then when you finish, sit quietly for several minutes with your eyes closed, and when you feel ready open your eyes.

Helpful tip: Make a note of where you feel the stress or anxiety most in your body. Is it in your head, chest or abdomen? Then on exhalation say to yourself, 'I release the tension in my ...'

Alternate Nostril Breathing

This is a great way to calm the mind. It can take a little time getting used to and the instructions may appear more complicated than they really are.

Make yourself comfortable in an upright-seated position. With your right hand, rest your pointer finger and middle finger between your eyebrows. Close your eyes and take a deep breath in and out through your nose. Close your right nostril with your right thumb. Inhale through the left nostril slowly and steadily then pause for a second. Now close your left nostril with your pointer finger on your right hand and release thumb from your right nostril. Exhale slowly through your right nostril pausing briefly before you inhale through the right nostril. Then use your thumb to close your right nostril and breathe out through your left nostril. This is one complete cycle. Begin with 5-10 rounds and gradually increase to longer rounds.

Try to be consistent with your inhales, pauses, and exhales. For example, try inhaling for a count of three, hold for three, exhaling for three, and holding for three. You can slowly increase your count as you refine your practice. Sit quietly for a few moments after you have finished.

A General Everyday Rule: Become more mindful about your breathing. Check in with your breath at different times of the day. Is it shallow and quick, or calm and relaxed? Or perhaps do you unconsciously holding your breath, which often occurs during moments of deep concentration? Deep breathing helps induce a 'relaxation response' as your nervous systems become more balanced. Regular elicitation of the relaxation response has been scientifically proven to be an effective treatment for a wide range of stress-related disorders.

16 October 2012
Robbed by Fear

My body is robbed by fear. Ever since the scan detected the liver cyst, confidence in my body has waned. I need to switch off my inner inquisitor to a 'wait and see' mode as opposed to its default 'worst-case scenario' position. But resistance is futile and I enter a panicked state. It's very difficult to quarantine fearful thoughts with traumatic health events still so fresh in my cellular memory.

I have put off making the appointment for as long as my nerves would hold out. In all probability I've been told it will be benign. But that's exactly what was said about my bowel polyp, until of course it turned out to be anything but!

The absence of certainty leads me on a path of 'what ifs' that soon spirals out of control, sending me into a mire of doubt, congealed by fear: a dangerous combination. I wish these scary, negative thoughts would exit my mind. I am so envious of people who don't appear overwhelmed by things, and take things in their stride. Why can't I be like them? Why do I cast an inquisitive glare and microscopically analyse every possible scenario? Rational thinking and faith are swiftly becoming a distant shadow. Inside I am like a feather swept up in the wind, unanchored and out of control.

The past year's traumatic memories flood my system. I summon the strength that supported and guided me through those difficult times, but it is nowhere to be found.

I procrastinate until I can procrastinate no longer and book the appointment. It's really out of my hands. Please God let everything be OK. What else can I wish for?

xoxo

Do you often leap to worst-case scenarios?

....

....

....

What things can you say to yourself to reassure and orient yourself towards a more positive mindset, free of fear?

....

....

....

19 October 2012

One hour prior to liver MRI. Note to myself

I promise to go with the flow and make changes in my life consistent with that mindset. I choose to be a healer: to heal others and myself using laughter yoga.

I relinquish doing academic work and instead embrace being a laughter professional, i.e. I emphasise heart over head. Thankfully we are in a position to do this, having now sold our house and not yet committed to another. I'm so grateful Danny is in full employment.

I will not look back. I will not have regrets.

If I ever have any doubts I will reflect on this entry. Time to move from survival mode, with my head barely skimming the water's edge, to live and thrive!

My energy has been running on a non-sustainable and debilitating energy source: nerves. I have been in denial about the cost of academic life on me. It once served me well, but now it's time for me to be my own power source: to follow my soul intention and heart's desire. I give up fighting for a life that isn't the right fit for me; giving until I've no more to give. I am ready to power up and know I will be supported in doing so.

I must not be afraid. Money will come, as will stability, and most importantly my health will be restored. I have been so swamped by everything, I have forgotten to have faith in my body's ability to restore health.

I choose *LIFE*

I choose to be a *HEALER*

I choose *VIBRANT HEALTH*

I choose *LAUGHTER.*

Let love be my guide and healer. Let it consume any residual fear lurking in the darkness. My future is bedazzling and bright, but like a spoilt child, I have given fear too much power. I choose the path of light and love.

X

If you could do whatever you wanted to do, what would you do?

....

....

....

How much power do you allow fear to have in preventing you from living the life of your dreams?

....

....

....

How can you eliminate fear?

....

....

....

Waiting Room Breathing Practice
(ideally 10 minutes)

Mindful breathing in a waiting room when there are so many distractions (internal and external) can be easier said than done, but this practice is ideal.

Numeric breathing

Close your eyes ideally and count your breaths from 1–10 and then back again, with each number being one complete breath. If you lose your place, just begin again. It's harder than you think.

It's a great distraction and definitely helps shift your worrying mind away from stressful thoughts. It works well in places filled with distractions, even workplaces.

29 October 2012

Anxiety

Creeping, seeping, forming a pathway of its own
In sync with my blood flow, running through my veins
Ebbing, weighing
Sinking deeper
Pulsating like a boa constrictor's stranglehold

Breathe
Breathe some more
Make it exit, breathe it out
This is not who I am
I do not want this to be a part of me
I yearn for peace
For calm to restore my tired, depleted body and exhausted mind

Just as you came I now beckon for you to depart
I acknowledge your presence
I accept things need to be different
Now give me space to make the changes I need
Restore peace to my body, mind and soul
Allow me to slowly open myself to change, to a different way
of being
Let me reclaim my body
Thanks for the message you have delivered to me
It's now time for you to leave.

Laugh Your Stress and Anxiety Away

Set a timer for one minute. Find a comfortable position to sit or lie, away from any disruptions or judgmental ears.

Close your eyes. Take a couple of deep breaths in and out. Start your timer and begin laughing. It might be helpful to think of something funny or simply laugh. Continue doing so for a full minute. It's amazing how long one minute can feel when you're laughing!

Take a further couple of deep breaths in and out before opening your eyes. How do you feel? Have you managed to laugh any of your anxiety, stress or frustration away?

Do this power laugh, stress-busting practice when you feel the need. You can even build it up to two or three minutes. Aside from being a brilliant mental health booster, it's also a great aerobic workout!

8 November 2012

To dream a dream

I've deserted you, journal, thinking perhaps I didn't need you as much as I do. Life went into full swing. I thought I had everything under control. I mean this was my 'recovery year'. I have empowered myself with so many positive thoughts and affirmations and worked through so much. I have basically bounced back, haven't I?

Yet in all honesty I haven't been bouncing anywhere. I've flopped here and flopped there, dotted with intermittent energy spurts that have delighted my inner being. I masquerade as a thriving success story but inside I am locked into survival mode, gasping for air.

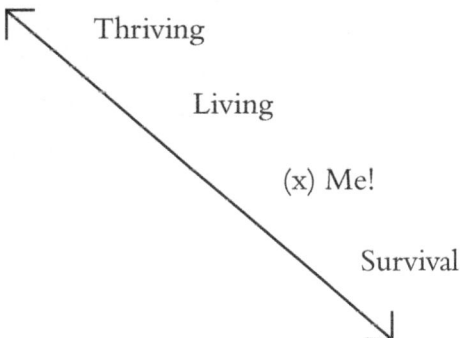

Denial is a strong concept, and whilst under its spell, I have convinced not only myself but also others of a different reality. Theoretically I was living my dream. The only problem is now my dream feels in part like someone else's. I am pining for a new one, but am not exactly sure what it looks like. Something's holding me back from fully committing and immersing myself in the laughter and writing world.

The moment I begin dreaming, the menacing voice in my head interjects saying, 'Seriously Ros, how could you throw it all away? So many people would 'die' for such an opportunity (there's a lesson in that word choice!) What about all those years studying? And now a permanent part-time lecturer position. This is clearly your destiny.'

But something definitely changed the day of my MRI. I had distracted myself with deep breathing in the waiting room, telling myself I would be OK, it would all be OK. However as I donned the white hospital gown and was ushered into the bed adjoining the MRI machine I began shaking violently. I was immobilised.

Disappearing into that tunnel, into the abyss, and having to lie perfectly still was the farthermost thing I could conceive of doing. I wanted to bolt the hell out of there. I almost did! It wasn't even the physical act of undergoing the MRI, as I'd had one before, it was the fear of what may be discovered. The technician halted my premature departure, reaching out for my hand and with a soothing voice comforted me for many moments before I hesitatingly conceded to give it a go. Through voiceover she continued reassuring me until both my own shaking and that of the MRI machine ceased.

In this case, thankfully, the liver cyst proved benign, but this whole episode served as a stark reminder of my mortality. Am I doing what I want to be doing? Have I achieved what I need to achieve? How many more scares will it take to get me onto my own path of fulfilment and satisfaction, where joy and laughter replace deadlines and stress? My physical body is my compass telling me I need to align with my True Self and I need to do it now.

What is your dream?

....
....
....

Are you on the right track?

....
....
....

What steps are you taking to make it come true?

....
....
....

Have you encountered any obstacles?

....
....
....

How did you deal with these?

....
....
....

13 November 2012
The bale of hay that broke the camel's back

The Jewish silly season has been and gone. I entertained and was entertained whilst immersed in social discourse, laughter and food, not only to savour, but also at this time of year, food for the soul. I love being social but a nagging feeling cautioned me not to overdo it, which was proving very challenging as everywhere I turned invitations were bestowed upon us. 'We'd love to have you for lunch,' 'Come to us to break the fast,' 'You have to come for dinner; it will only be something small.' I found it hard to refuse such kindness, especially when three other family members were always keen to go out and be fed. My inner, rational voice piped up, 'I'd just have to feed them anyway, and after all these are festive meals.'

Slouched on an enticingly comfy couch at a friend's house before one of the many formal lunch proceedings, all I wanted to do was kick my shoes off and not move an inch for a very long time. Yet, like a wind-up doll in chronic need of winding, I shuffled to the dining table, feigning enthusiasm and energy for the conversation that ensued. As much as I was present, I was absent. I had a feeling I would pay for this.

After many more dinner rounds, together with mounting assignments that were refusing to mark themselves, lead weights now replaced normal functioning in my legs, and my heart began strangely fluttering and palpitating erratically. Breathe … breathe … don't worry. I hear you! Disquietingly, during the past couple of weeks, I had bumped into three friends and acquaintances who'd recently had serious heart incidents, two major, and one that happily transpired to be nothing more than a scare.

With my heart still in flutters, I decided it was high time to face my fears and visit my GP. When I entered her room a student doctor was present. She asked if I minded whether she stayed for my consultation, uncharacteristically I said that *'Yes, I did mind.'* The last thing I wanted was to discuss my current stress levels and pattering heart in front of a student, given that, in large part, the way I felt was due to my student load. Oh, the ironies!

Exit the student doctor.

I then was able to freely bemoan about my student load and how I felt like a phoney lecturing in health promotion whilst feeling like the person least invested in my own. I also told her about the panic attack I'd had on the MRI machine, and even though, thank God, the cyst had proved benign, my nerves were still very much on edge.

She looked me deep in the eyes with a gaze that penetrated far into my soul and said I should resign and focus on my laughter work. 'You love doing that, don't you?' I did and wished it were that simple, I said, to which she responded, 'You really need to, for you.'

She then handed me blood test forms and a request for a 24-hour heart monitor halter. She also relayed it was not uncommon for people to have a delayed stress response, i.e. post-traumatic stress, often appearing 12 or so months after the event. I felt comforted knowing that, as unpleasant as all this was, it was not an unreasonable or unexpected occurrence. Dare I say it could almost be construed within the realms of normalcy?

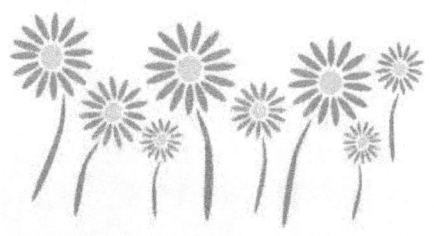

Can you recall a particular incident in your life that led to a downward spiral or catapulting of events?

....

....

....

Reflecting on this time, what was the most important lesson you learnt?

....

....

....

16 November 2012
What is stress?

Today I have been thinking about stress: a catch-all word, not even a phrase. What does it really mean? Undoubtedly it involves a withering of internal peace and calm caused by pressure and tension. Yet it's a term so generalised that it can be used to describe a litany of woes and concerns. Surely this is a deficiency in the English language? It's impossible for one word to describe so many feelings. 'I'm feeling stressed' is a phrase I have uttered ever since childhood when things, for lack of a better word, were stressful. How can you respond to and remedy a stressful situation if you're not really sure what you're dealing with?

Time to deconstruct this bully. What's the trigger? Ill health, anxiety, workload, frustration, financial pressure, lack of choices or control, family-life imbalance and ineffective communication? Sometimes, stress cannot be pinned down to a single factor but to a combination of several causes that might be creating an overload. What type of stress response is occurring? Anxiety, emotional pain, general overwhelm, fear, panic?

Although it's undeniably helpful to identify the sources of stress and the types of reaction it leads to, this exercise only paints part of the picture. I'm curious, what factors affect our ability to cope with stress? I know there are times when my internal coping mechanisms are bolstered, no matter what's going on in the external environment. My sense of humour kicks in and I feel like I can take anything on. At other times however, the humour is booted out along with my resilience.

This afternoon, I set out on a meditative quest to explore the sensations of stress within me. I had not been able to attain the answers I had hoped for in my conscious state, but I knew I would be able to sit with these thoughts more deeply, insightfully and expansively, in a meditative state. After slowing and deepening my breath, I tapped into any internal disquiet—the unease. I speculated at just how much distance lay between unease and disease. I began observing this thing called stress, pulsating like a jellyfish's tentacles encircling my gut, heart, chest and throat, and gently tugging at the muscles around my throat and jaw. The sensations became more dense and solid as their amorphous bodies spilled out inside my head.

I allowed myself to feel these vivid sensations for just a while longer before summoning my breath and a gentle smile to dissolve this menacing alien. I breathed in newness, serenity and light, and exhaled unease, angst and darkness. I don't know how long this exchange continued, but after a period of time lightness descended throughout my whole being. For a moment or two longer I sat in peace and stillness before opening my eyes.

What a powerful meditation session. It may not have wiped the stress-slate clean, but something has shifted, and not just that big amorphous blob! The edge of my anxiety has softened and my heart rhythm has settled. I'm so grateful today I wasn't *too busy* to meditate!

Where do you feel stress in your body? (jaws, chest, gut, heart, head, legs?)

....

....

....

Do you have a daily stress - busting ritual? (Meditation, working - out, going for a walk, deep breathing) If not, think of something you can do to keep stress at bay.

17 November 2012

What you focus on grows

Today a word find puzzle in the newspaper caught my attention. With pen at hand I eagerly embarked on this welcome distraction, but my enthusiasm soon waned. It was simplistic and non-stimulating. So with a penchant for love hearts and desire to be more wellbeing-focused, I went to the task of designing my own. So many words came to mind a deluge of positivity. Such fun!

Wellbeing Word Find

```
          N E C K                 J E H Y
      I J J M O W             R J O V M S
    C X A A S P C R         U M M R W G S Z
  I O N K T Q F O B V N K T O E O N E M E
F N M Y H F H V Q W R R T M C S H I N E Z E
U C S P T R O P P U S E M N S O P B L I J W E J
U O F A E T Y W C Q T M R X R M E V I P L D Y U
R N N S M O D E E R F U V M O M C I M P A B H Y
H T S S E N L U F D N I M R E U T I S A U C T D
U R P I Y W V L O V E M D I X N Q R Y H G U A R
E O W O A N V P E A C E D V C I T I K B H C P E
  L D N C X T G A B U N D A N C E Q M S T G M
  K M S I L A U D I V I D N I A B E L M E G E
    Q U M Q W E C N A L A B D T D H S C R G
      P I H S D N E I R F W R I I Q D M U
        F T I U Y K P S O Y T O T U S Y
          S E Y V O I L P A P N W I S
            U A Z K F K T A E O M H
              R E O X I W P C I Z
                F U O B P U T E
                  N M K H P W
                    Z G O Q
                      J G
```

ABUNDANCE
BALANCE
COMMUNICATION
COMPASSION
CONTROL
EMPATHY
EMPOWERMENT
FLOW
FREEDOM
FRIENDSHIP
HAPPINESS
INDIVIDUALISM
LAUGHTER
LOVE
MEDITATION
MINDFULNESS
OPTIMISM
PEACE
RESPECT
SMILING
SPACE
SUPPORT

20 November 2012

My Epiphany Moment

I was freaking out; my heart rhythm was all over the place. In the wee hours of the morning I calmly told it to relax and slow down, but it was racing away, and no matter how hard I tried, I couldn't catch it.

I was fitted with a 24-hour heart monitor causing even more anxiety as wires were strapped onto my fretful body and an eco-cardiogram conducted. Today of all days I was beginning a laughter yoga research program, the Laugh out Loud (LOL) Project, with a colleague from my university. Preparations for this project had begun prior to any personal connection to a bowel resection or the likes.

This was week one in a 6-week program to investigate the effect of a 30-minute laughter session on residents' blood pressure and heart rate. Oh the ironies! My heart monitored simultaneously to participants. That was most definitely not part of the original plan.

I chose my wardrobe carefully, opting for a high-collared buttoned shirt with extra length to obscure the wires and 'Sony Walkman' monitor.

Before I entered the aged care facility I gently smacked my cheeks, tricking them into a healthy glow. Feeling twice my age I immediately felt right at home. They say laughter is the best medicine and I was certainly testing the theory. I mustered a smile and channelled some degree of enthusiasm before introducing myself and explaining the unique concept of laughter yoga. Here I refer to it as laughter exercises or laughter activities as yoga terminology would just be confusing.

The session began with some deep-breathing exercises. They

appeared to be coping well, but the deep breaths were tugging at my heartstrings. As for stretching, my mainframe felt like fossilised bone. I demonstrated additional breathing techniques but stopped short of fully extending my arms as I was self-conscious of wires poking out and worried the weighty monitor would dislodge. I demonstrated the first laugh, tapping our bodies awake with laughter tapping, before a series of vocal and coordination-based laughs. We imbibed laughter cocktails and ran a laughter marathon. I was constantly observing and gauging how they were managing this surprisingly aerobic exercise. Today I included myself in this monitoring process and slowed things down as the need arose.

We continued for a further 15 minutes, allowing time to catch our breath. I asked one of my favourite questions, 'Why do you like to laugh?' Over the years I have been asking many groups this particular question and found the most popular response is, 'Because it makes me happy.' Today was no exception. Even one of the ladies who suffered from dementia and had lost the ability to verbally communicate responded with a smile. Just seeing and hearing their responses warmed my heart and put a smile on my face. In all these years I have yet to meet someone who didn't like to laugh.

The session went well. It certainly was the best I had felt in weeks, and judging by the glint in their eyes and chatter after the session, it seemed to have been an all-round success. Immediately after the session one of the nursing staff monitored their blood pressure and turned to me with a look of concern, unsure whether it should have been higher or lower than the readings they took before the session. I responded 'ideally lower', whereby she heaved a sigh of relief as in most residents blood pressure was indeed lower.

That night even with the intermittent prodding of wires, so much stress had dissipated that I slept relatively soundly. Naturally, I was not sorry to farewell the heart monitor the next morning and relieved that during those past 24 hours I'd had several heart irregularities—which might seem a strange thing to write but having gone to the effort of having a heart monitor I wanted any misbehavings noted. Of course all I really wanted was for it to return to peaceful beating and not give it a second thought. I was also curious. Would the monitor detect any decrease in heart rate during those 30-minutes? Not that I needed any scientific proof. Within myself I knew how much more relaxed I felt.

The day after, still feeling like a wrung out rag, I was scheduled to facilitate a laughter session at a prestigious girls' school. At the time of booking several months prior, I had been so excited to get my foot in the door. Now I wondered how I would get it out. I spent the morning resting my eyes, breathing deeply and psyching myself up to muster the energy I would need to match that of 120 excitable 17-year-old girls. 'Oh well,' I said to myself once again, 'I can do it. In any case I've got no choice.' I then attempted to extricate myself from the living room couch—my 'home away from home' within my home.

Both the size of the group and that of the hall were too large to rely on my voice alone for this session, and so on arrival I requested a microphone. A sound technician was summoned to feed a wire through my shirt and secure a sound box to the outside of my trouser pocket; the very same pocket where a heart monitor box had rested just a day ago and the same part of my chest where its wires had crisscrossed.

Then silence. Time stood still as the heavens opened up and a bright light streamed down onto the stage. An imaginary voice resonated, 'If you continue the way you have been doing, you will be in for a life of stress and ill health. Choose laughter and all will be well!'

I was almost tempted to ask the teacher at my side if she too had heard the voice, but of course it had been in my head. Miraculously the session went well. 'I got away with it,' I thought to myself.

Over the years I had received several signs relating to laughter and the significant role it would play in my life, but none like this. This was an epiphany moment. I was so excited. I had always wanted an epiphany; I just never imagined how it would happen or what exactly it would be about. This one I couldn't ignore. I knew what I had to do. I had to orient my life around laughter, not the other way around. The only way I could do that was to take the bold step and resign from my energy-sapping teaching position. In this epiphany moment I made a promise to choose laughter, to choose happiness and to be well. I'd had a taste of the alternative and it was 100%, most definitely NOT for me.

What an amazing day! What an amazing week! I feel so liberated and with a heightened sense of euphoria for the present moment as well as the journey ahead.

Thinking about it, laughter really is an innate super-power. It's just sometimes we need to remind ourselves it is actually there for the taking and the sharing. A common language we share with all other members of the globe, laughter and smiling occur naturally from the earliest stages of our development. I recall the all-encompassing smile on two-day-old Zak that prompted an unscheduled name change from Gabriel to Yitzchak, stemming from the Hebrew root for to laugh, "Litzchok". And no, I was 100 percent sure it was not wind! He was going to be a laugher.

These past couple of days, although in all probability it has been months or even years, have brazenly shown me that laughter has to be my compass to guide me on life's journey: to make me more resilient, fill my life and the lives of others with joy and vitality. That's my wish: To be supported on my laughter path.

xoxo

And Ros lived happily ever laughter
The End.

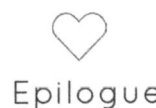

Epilogue

17 June 2016 marked five years since my bowel resection. For people who have had cancer, five years is very much a psychological marker – a time to fully exhale. Even though within myself I knew all was well, I was elated to hear the specialist's words, 'You're cured'. Although at the time I recall being slightly bemused by his word choice – for some reason in my mind 'cured' was a term more synonymous with salmon or meat, rather than my own body. I much prefer healed: far more empowering and wholesome. I can't say I was sorry to see the backside (pun intended) of regular checkups or annual CT scans, but I am very accepting of precautionary bi-annual colonoscopies.

I had always intended to publish these journals as a book, however for a range of reasons paused before taking the plunge. I was wary of going back into an 'illness or cancer' space. I wanted to immerse myself in laughter, mindfulness and wellness to avoid a fleeting concern: that the bowel cancer may define me. I also became my dad's main support, as he succumbed to Alzheimer's disease following the sad passing of his beloved, my mum.

When the timing felt right at the end of 2014 I resigned from my formal teaching position to develop and deliver laughter, mindfulness and wellbeing programs. I was prompted to revisit the journals after a series of shock diagnoses of close friends and relatives with assorted illnesses. Having not laid my eyes on the journals for a couple of years I was relieved and delighted to discover how filled with love, laughter and optimism they were. I was also amazed that without conscious awareness, the MORE

LAUGHTER Wellbeing framework I developed was very much informed by these experiences, as you will see:

M indfulness
O ptimistic style
R elationships
E mpathy & compassion (for self and others)

L aughter
A ppreciation and gratitude
U nique (what makes you unique?)
G oals
H elping others
T eamwork
E ndorphin boosters
R elaxation

Up until recently I have largely hidden my experience with bowel cancer from public. When I have divulged this, many people look at me in surprise, as I seemingly don't fit the mould of a typical bowel cancer candidate. Now a cushion of time acts as a buffer and I feel ready for the journey ahead.

Every day I am grateful the bowel cancer was detected early. I practice gratitude and mindfulness daily using many of the techniques outlined in this book. I still need to take the odd 'pyjama day' and at times become frustrated by my body's physical limitations, but overall I know I am truly blessed.

My life is filled with joy, love and laughter thanks to my beautiful family and friends. For this I am eternally grateful.

In love and laughter,

Ros.

References

p.9   Gawler, I., The Mind that Changes Everything, Brolga Publishing,

p.18   Kataria, M. Laughter Yoga International http://laughteryoga.org, 1999

p.19   Doidge, N., The Brain That Changes Itself, James H. Silberman Books, 2007 (Scribe Australia 2008)

p.87   Lyubomirsky, S., Sheldon, K. M., & Schkade, D. (2005). Pursuing happiness: The architecture of sustainable change. Review of General Psychology, 9, 111-131.

p.149   Seligman, M.E.P., Authentic Happiness: Using the New Positive Psychology to Realize Your Potential for Lasting Fulfillment. New York: Free Press. 2004

p.214   Temoshok, L., Unraveling the 'Type C' Connection: Is There a Cancer Personality? Implications for Prevention & Recovery (http://www.healingcancer.info/ebook/lydia-temoshok)

p.215   Maté, G. (2003). When the Body Says No – Exploring the Stress Disease Connection, John Wiley & sons, New Jersey.

Laughing at Cancer

Ros Ben Moshe

ISBN: 9781925367843   Qty

            RRP   AU$24.99 .....

Postage within Australia   AU$5.00   .....

                 TOTAL* $_____

                 * All prices include GST

Name: ....

Address: ....

....

Phone: ....

Email: ....

Payment: [ ] Money Order   [ ] Cheque   [ ] MasterCard   [ ]Visa

Cardholder's Name:...

Credit Card Number: ....

Signature:...

Expiry Date: ....

Allow 7 days for delivery.

Payment to: Marzocco Consultancy (ABN 14 067 257 390)
                  PO Box 12544
                  A'Beckett Street, Melbourne, 8006
                  Victoria, Australia
                  admin@brolgapublishing.com.au

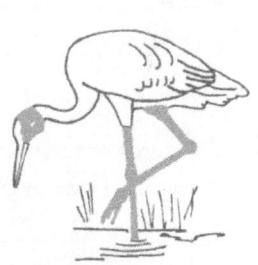

Be Published

Publish through a successful publisher.
Brolga Publishing is represented through:
• **National** book trade distribution, including sales, marketing & distribution through Dennis Jones and Associates Australia.
  • **International** book trade distribution to
    • The United Kingdom
    • North America
    • Sales representation in South East Asia
• **Worldwide e-Book distribution**

For details and inquiries, contact:
Brolga Publishing Pty Ltd
PO Box 12544
A'Beckett St VIC 8006

Phone: 0414 608 494
markzocchi@brolgapublishing.com.au
ABN: 46 063 962 443
(Email for a catalogue request)